ASTHMA

ASTHMA

The Biography

Mark Jackson

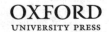

OXFORD
UNIVERSITY PRESS

OXFORD
UNIVERSITY PRESS

Great Clarendon Street, Oxford OX2 6DP

Oxford University Press is a department of the University of Oxford.
It furthers the University's objective of excellence in research, scholarship,
and education by publishing worldwide in

Oxford New York

Auckland Cape Town Dar es Salaam Hong Kong Karachi
Kuala Lumpur Madrid Melbourne Mexico City Nairobi
New Delhi Shanghai Taipei Toronto

With offices in

Argentina Austria Brazil Chile Czech Republic France Greece
Guatemala Hungary Italy Japan Poland Portugal Singapore
South Korea Switzerland Thailand Turkey Ukraine Vietnam

Oxford is a registered trade mark of Oxford University Press
in the UK and in certain other countries

Published in the United States
by Oxford University Press Inc., New York

British Library Cataloguing in Publication Data
Data available

Library of Congress Cataloging-in-Publication Data
Jackson, Mark, 1959–
Asthma : the biography / Mark Jackson.
p. ; cm.—(Biographies of disease)
Includes bibliographical references and index.
ISBN 978-0-19-923795-1 (hardback : alk. paper)
1. Asthma—History. I. Title. II. Series: Biographies of disease (Oxford, England)
[DNLM: 1. Asthma—history. WF 11.1 J13a 2009]
RC591.J315 2009
616.2'38—dc22   2009026412

Typeset by SPI Publisher Services, Pondicherry, India
Printed in Great Britain
on acid-free paper by
Clays Ltd, St Ives plc

ISBN 978-0-19-923795-1

1 3 5 7 9 10 8 6 4 2

For Ciara, Riordan, and Conall

L'amour c'est l'espace et le temps rendus sensibles au cœur.
Marcel Proust, *La Prisonnière*

ACKNOWLEDGEMENTS

Unlike asthma, this book has a relatively straightforward history. Approximately two years ago, Bill and Helen Bynum asked me to contribute a volume on asthma to a new edited series entitled 'Biographies of Disease', to be published by Oxford University Press. Since it seemed an excellent idea, I agreed, and the book was born. I am deeply grateful to Bill and Helen for their constructive, and astonishingly swift and generous, advice and support throughout the process of preparing the manuscript. I am also indebted to Latha Menon from Oxford University Press for her careful coordination and management of the project.

The research on which the book is based was funded by the Wellcome Trust, and I am grateful both for the Trust's financial support and for the advice and friendship of key figures within the Trust, particularly Mark Walport, Clare Matterson, Tony Woods, and Liz Shaw. Since the chronological and geographical range of the subject extended well beyond my usual terms of historical reference, I am afraid that I relied on the generosity of many colleagues, who shared their work, time, and ideas in order to facilitate my access to the previously hidden depths of ancient and modern, Western and Eastern, histories of medicine. In particular, I would like to thank Guy Attewell, Sanjoy Bhattacharya, Siam Bhayro, Roberta Bivins, Jeremy Black, Maarten Bode, Tse Wen Chang, Philip van der Eijk, Alison Finch, Ali Haggett, Rhodri Hayward, Harry Hendrick, Carla Keirns, Ian Gregg, Tak Lee, Vivienne Lo, Gregg Mitman, Glen Needham,

Carol Parry, David van Sickle, Matthew Smith, Akihito Suzuki, and John Wilkins. I am also grateful to staff in the inter-library loan section of the University of Exeter Library for obtaining copies of otherwise inaccessible articles and books, and to Asthma UK for allowing me access to the early records of the Asthma Research Council.

I am grateful to the following sources for the illustrations and permission to reproduce them: Figure 1: http://commons/ wikimedia.org/wiki/Image:Marcel_Proust_1900.jpg; Figures 2, 3, 4, 5, 7, 8, and 10 are reproduced courtesy of the Wellcome Library, London; Figure 6 is from Clyde Henderson Thompson, 'Marin Marais, 1656–1728' (Ph.D. thesis, University of Michigan, 1957); Figures 9 and 11 are reproduced courtesy of the Advertising Archives, London; Figure 12 is provided by the Centre for the Study of Cartoons and Caricature, Templeman Library, University of Kent, copyright Mirrorpix, 1958, reproduced by permission of Mirrorpix; Figures 13 and 15 are Crown copyright, reproduced from the Lung and Asthma Information Agency Factsheets 97/3 and 2001/1, http://www.sghms.ac.uk/ depts/laia/laia.htm; Figure 14 is a scanning electron micrograph of an American house dust mite reproduced by kind permission of Glen Needham, Acarology Laboratory, the Ohio State University, Columbus, Ohio. I have made every effort to contact all copyright holders. If proper acknowledgement has not been made, I ask the copyright holders to contact the publishers.

Of course, my heart belongs to Siobhán, who breathed fresh life into me many years ago and who will always be the fulcrum of my world. The book is dedicated, however, to our three children, Ciara, Riordan, and Conall, who have so beautifully filled our space and time.

CONTENTS

LIST OF ILLUSTRATIONS

PROLOGUE

Il n'y a pas de maladies; il n'y a que des malades.
French aphorism

I n a brief letter written to his devoted mother in 1900, the French novelist Marcel Proust complained that the previous day he had suffered from an 'attack of asthma of unbelievable violence and tenacity', which had obliged him to spend all night on his feet in spite of extreme tiredness. Such episodes of acutely debilitating asthma were not unusual for Proust during this period of his life. In another intimate note to his mother, dated 26 August 1901, Proust described how, having travelled to Versailles to visit some distant relatives, he had been 'seized with a horrifying attack of asthma, so that I didn't know what to do or where to hide myself'. A few days later, his misery continued unabated:

> Yesterday after I wrote to you I had an attack of asthma and incessant running at the nose, which obliged me to walk all doubled up and light anti-asthma cigarettes at every tobacconist's I passed, etc. And what's worse, I haven't been able to go to bed till midnight, after endless fumigations, and it's three or fours hours after a real summer attack, an unheard of thing for me. Such a thing has never happened outside the usual season for my attacks.[1]

Marcel Proust was born in Paris on 10 July 1871, at a moment of widespread political unrest in France following the disastrous Paris Commune earlier that year. His Roman Catholic father, Dr Adrien Proust (1834–1903), was a prominent doctor who had chosen to remain in Paris to treat those wounded during street battles between the revolutionary National Guard and the Versailles army. Renowned particularly for his work on cholera and public health, Adrien was one of the founders of the International Office of Hygiene and the co-author of a treatise on neurasthenia, in which he suggested that maternal over-affection might cause nervous diseases. Significantly, Marcel was deeply attached to his Jewish mother, Jeanne (née Weill), who remained his closest carer and confidante, and to whom he wrote almost daily messages, until her death in 1905.[2]

Marcel Proust suffered his first severe attack of asthma when he was 9 years old, while out walking with his family in the Bois de Boulogne. From that moment, asthma and hay fever, along with many other recurrent complaints such as insomnia, indigestion, back pain, headaches, dizziness, and fatigue, began to plague his life: during early adulthood Proust became a chronic invalid, often confined to his room, and indeed his bed, as he

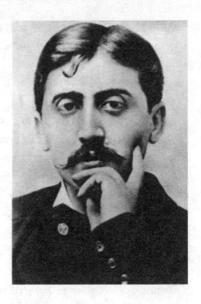

1. Marcel Proust, 1871–1922.

attempted to cope with persistent ill health and maintain his intellectual creativity. Having graduated in law and philosophy in the early 1890s, Proust published his first book *Les Plaisirs et les jours* in 1896 and began work on *Jean Santeuil*, which was published only in 1952. After the death of his father in 1903, and of his mother two years later, Proust's health declined further. In 1906, following the publication of his celebrated translation of Ruskin, he retreated to his Parisian apartment at 102, Boulevard Haussmann to compose his finest work, *À la recherche du temps perdu*, translated into English as *In Search of Lost Time*. Comprising seven volumes, three of which were published after his death by his younger brother Robert, this sequence of novels exploring interlocking themes of space, time, memory, love, and jealousy established Proust as perhaps the greatest modern French writer.

As Proust's letters to his mother and his friends testify, asthma was a constant companion until his death in 1922. Violent attacks of coughing, gasping, and choking dominated his life. In 1907, in a letter to his loyal friend Madame Straus, on whom he later based the character of the Duchesse de Guermantes, Proust explained why he had not been in contact: 'And ever since that moment up to today (and until I don't know when in the future), I haven't stopped choking and having incessant attacks. And that is why, although you were in my thoughts practically all day long, I haven't written; I haven't had the courage to take up my pen.' Similarly, in 1920, he wrote to his fellow author Marcel Boulenger, describing how he had 'been gasping for breath so continuously (incessant attacks of asthma for several days) that it is not very easy for me to write'.[3]

In addition to demonstrating the enormous impact of asthma on his life, Proust's correspondence provides evidence of the range of contemporary theories about the causes of asthma. According to Proust, episodes of asthma were most frequently precipitated by physical triggers such as dust, flowers, cold, damp, odours, certain foods, and changes in the weather. Indeed, his anxiety to avoid exposure to harmful pollutants and variable environmental conditions not only led him to remove gas from, and forbid cooking in, his apartment, but also encouraged him to construct a cork-lined bedroom that effectively protected him from pollen and perfume. Proust's compulsive reading of medical texts also prompted him to consider alternative and less conventional explanations for his asthma; in 1901, having read Édouard Brissaud's work on asthma, the preface to which had been written by his father, Proust feared that his troubles might be caused by threadworms, and asked his brother, who was a urologist, to recommend an appropriate enema as treatment.[4]

Proust was also aware that his asthma and hay fever were exacerbated by psychological and emotional factors. In a letter to his mother in 1904, for example, he reported that he had gone 'to bed in a state of great agitation, in consequence of which, I think, I had an attack of asthma. I went to sleep all the same, but had dreams of not being able to breathe, and at last woke up.'[5] Proust's family and friends were more critical. Much to Proust's dismay, they regarded many of his illnesses as the product of nervousness, indolence, and hypochondria, believing him to be a 'malade imaginaire'.[6] In a letter written to his mother in 1899 from Evian-les-Bains, a popular health resort on the southern shores of Lake Geneva, Proust dejectedly contrasted his own experience of the perils of asthma with his father's dismissive interpretation of his illness:

> By the way, as they wanted to bring me back in the car, Constantin said it was all in my imagination that cold air was bad for me, because Papa told everyone that there was nothing wrong with me and that my asthma was purely imaginary. I know only too well when I wake here in the morning that it is very real.[7]

Proust experimented with a wide variety of treatments in an attempt to alleviate or cure his asthma. While living at home before his parents died, he would retreat to a designated smoking room, in which he smoked medicated cigarettes or burned and inhaled Espic, Legras, or Escouflaire powders, all of which contained stramonium, an ancient remedy derived from thorn apple or jimson weed; his letters are replete with references to regular 'fumigations' with these patent remedies and other substances, such as carbolic acid. In addition, he was prescribed morphine, opium, caffeine, and iodine, had his nose cauterized as a child, adopted a milk diet, and attempted to avoid pollen and fumes either by living largely in isolation or by escaping to coastal or mountainous resorts, initially with his grandmother or mother, where the air was supposedly cleaner and healthier. On several occasions, particularly after his asthma had worsened following his mother's death, Proust sought advice from clinicians who specialized in treating nervous diseases, such as Édouard Brissaud (1852–1909) and Joseph Babinski (1857–1932), and spent six weeks in isolation in a clinic run by Paul Sollier (1861–1938) in Boulogne-sur-Seine.[8] Such efforts to relieve his distress proved in vain. Asthma remained an integral part of his life, leading some of his doctors and certain historians to suggest either that ultimately Proust did not want to be cured or, as his housekeeper Céleste Albaret admitted, that his asthma served a psychological or practical purpose, allowing him to avoid military service or to shun society in order to write:

> I think the truth is that he used even his illness as a further means of shutting himself up in his work and cutting himself off from the world outside. He wasn't afraid of illness. The only thing he feared was dying before he had finished his work. So he did all he could to erect as many walls as possible around himself.[9]

Asthma not only dominated Proust's daily existence but also infected his literature, colouring his characters and, according to some critics, even dictating his syntax.[10] As Proust himself acknowledged, there were close correlations between the description and analysis of events in his major literary work, *In Search of Lost Time*, and the details of his own life and the lives of those around him: the fictional narrator was also named Marcel and suffered from a similar range of symptoms, including periodic shortness of breath. Shaped by his familiarity with the latest medical theories as well as by his own experiences of illness, Proust's creative writings offer additional insights into both contemporary strategies for moderating asthma attacks and broader social perceptions of the disease. Proust's portrayal of asthma was characteristically astute. In the first volume of the series, *Du côté de chez Swann*, translated either as *Swann's Way* or as *The Way by Swann's*, Proust not only acknowledged the possibility that asthma could affect the working classes, contrary to contemporary medical opinion, but also recognized the manner in which a tendency to asthma could be exploited by others for personal gain: the kitchen maid was eventually forced by the cook to leave her employment because she was ordered repeatedly and deliberately to prepare asparagus, which precipitated her asthma.[11] Equally, in the second volume, *In the Shadow of Young Girls in Flower*, in addition to recounting popular medical approaches to treating asthma, Proust hinted at the manner in which asthmatics themselves could, on occasions, embroider their symptoms to influence those around them:

> For years I had suffered from attacks of shortness of breath; and our doctor, despite the disapproval of my grandmother, who was convinced I would go to an alcoholic's early grave, had recommended that, in addition to the caffeine already prescribed as an aid to my breathing, I should have a drink of beer, champagne or brandy each time I felt an attack coming on. The 'euphoria' brought on by the alcohol would, he said, 'nip it in the bud'. Rather than conceal the state of breathlessness I was in, I was often obliged almost to exaggerate it, before my grandmother would allow me to have such a drink.[12]

Marcel Proust's traumatic experiences and literary portrayals of asthma were clearly contingent, shaped not only by the peculiar circumstances of his life but also by the composition and boundaries of medical knowledge at the time. His interpretation of his illness as the product of a complex mix of constitutional factors, exposure to external environmental triggers, and challenging personal situations reflected contemporary medical approaches to the causes and manifestations of asthma. The diverse treatment regimes that he adopted, often without success, also mirrored both the wide range of conflicting therapies regularly advertised for the condition and his own obsessions with his physical and mental state of health. Equally, attempts by his peers (and indeed by historians) to explain Proust's many afflictions, as well as his barely concealed homosexuality, in terms of his close attachment to, and over-dependence on, his mother, can be understood as the product of a particular time and place. From this perspective, Proust's asthma was both historically and personally specific.

At the same time, however, Proust constitutes the archetypal asthmatic, whose breathlessness and discomfort echo across space and time. Proust's intimate descriptions of his symptoms—'an asthmatic never knows if he will be able to breathe', he wrote to the novelist André Gide in 1919[13]—bear striking similarities both to ancient Greek and medieval accounts of asthma many centuries earlier and to recent surveys suggesting that, at the turn of the millennium, many asthmatics continue to suffer from severe attacks that prevent them from speaking or make them fear for their lives. Thus, while medical understandings of, and treatments for, asthma have often shifted dramatically across time, the physical manifestations, existential impact, descriptive language, and symbolic significance of asthma have remained comparatively constant.

Recognizing that both medical understandings and patient experiences of asthma have been marked by continuity as well as by change, this book traces the complex story of asthma from the first recorded use of the term almost three thousand years ago to current accounts of the disease at the dawn of the twenty-first century. Chapter 1 explores classical approaches to asthma, and particularly the prominent focus on phlegm, not only in the ancient and medieval Western worlds, but also in the traditional Eastern medical systems prevalent in ancient China and India. Chapter 2 analyses the manner in which ancient accounts of asthma were gradually challenged from the late sixteenth century through to the mid-nineteenth century, in particular tracing emergent debates about the role of nervous bronchospasm in asthmatic paroxysms. Chapter 3 examines the links that were gradually forged between asthma and allergies, the proliferation of specialist asthma clinics, and the elaboration of novel pharmacological and psychodynamic approaches to the treatment of asthma during the first half of the twentieth century. The final chapter surveys international patterns of disease and death from asthma during the decades following the Second World War and evaluates contemporary anxieties about the spreading socioeconomic, political, and personal impact of asthma in the modern, globalized world.

Juxtaposing scientific and clinical accounts with the more intimate reflections of asthmatics themselves, the following pages constitute not only the biography of a particular disease but also a chronicle of the suffering, fears, and hopes of people with asthma, both past and present.

I

∞∞∞

CLASSICAL ASTHMA

Its onslaught is of very brief duration—like a squall, it is generally over within the hour. One could hardly, after all, expect anyone to keep on drawing his last breath for long, could one? I have suffered every kind of unpleasant or dangerous physical complaint, but none is worse than this. Not surprising, for anything else is just an illness, while this is gasping out your life-breath.

Seneca, *Epistulae Morales ad Lucilium*, c. AD 62–5

A sthma has a long history. The term itself derives from an ancient Greek word, ασθμα, which first appeared in Homer's epic poem *The Iliad*, composed in the seventh or eighth century BC. At the start of Book 15, Zeus awakes to discover the Trojan army dispersed by the Greeks, and the Trojan leader, Hector, 'lying on the plain, while about him sat his comrades, and he was gasping with painful breath [*asthmati*], distraught in mind, and vomiting blood'. Later in the same book, Homer describes Hector's recovery, in which his 'gasping [*asthma*] and his sweat had ceased'.[1]

Homer's choice of the word 'asthma' to denote the laboured breathing, panting, and gasping induced by exertion was reinforced by other ancient writers. Both the Greek playwright Aeschylus (525–456 BC) and the Greek lyrical poet Pindar (522–443 BC) used the term in similar ways in the fifth century BC. In *The Persians, Eumenides*, and *The Seven against Thebes*, Aeschylus employed the term 'asthma' to describe the panting or breathlessness that could be generated either by fury or by battle exhaustion. For Pindar, in his *Nemean Odes*, asthma denoted both the convulsive gasps of Castor, who lay close to death having been stabbed by Idas, and the 'panting bodies' of wild boars slain by Achilles. A century later, Plato (428–348 BC) exploited this Homeric tradition in his influential philosophical reflections on political theory and justice, *The Republic*, written in approximately 360 BC. For Plato, asthma carried two meanings. On the one hand, he used it to refer to the 'panting' helplessness of wealthy, indolent men in the face of battle; on the other hand, it also signified, in metaphorical terms, the limited honour or courage that often paralysed political action, 'as it were from lack of breath' (*asthmatos*).[2]

Yet intriguingly, while popular usage of the term persisted in classical Greece and Rome, by Plato's time asthma had obtained a more specific medical meaning. In the works of Hippocrates and others from the fifth century BC, asthma had begun to constitute not merely a generic sign of extreme physical exhaustion or moral weakness, but also a relatively distinct form of pathology with its own symptoms, causes, prognosis, and treatments. In the treatises attributed to Hippocrates, for example, there are at least forty-seven references to asthma as a type of difficult breathing, many of which attempt to account for the geographical and demographic distribution and the individual experiences of asthma in terms of environmental factors and personal disposition. It was largely this clinical description of asthma that was consolidated and transmitted by medical authors in the ancient world and subsequently adopted and adapted by medieval scholars.

This predominantly Western tradition, however, was not the only, nor indeed necessarily the earliest, formulation of laboured breathing as a medical condition requiring discrete management and the application of specific herbal remedies. The causes of, and possible treatments for, noisy breathing and coughing, symptoms that were subsequently assimilated under the term 'asthma', were discussed not only by early Chinese authors, such as Shen Nung and Huang Di, nearly three thousand years BC, but also by āyurvedic practitioners in India, by ancient Egyptian doctors, and by Japanese and Korean physicians in the pre-modern periods. Indeed, as will become apparent, many modern Western therapeutic approaches to asthma, such as the administration of ephedrine or the inhalation of stramonium, were originally derived from ancient Eastern remedies.

Ancient accounts

According to legend, Hippocrates was born on the Greek island of Kos in approximately 460 BC. His interest in medicine may have come initially from his family: his mother was reputedly a midwife and his father and grandfather were physicians. However, Hippocrates also undertook more formal medical training, possibly under the tutelage of the physician Herodicus, at the *asklepieion* (or healing temple) in Kos. Having rapidly acquired a reputation for both erudite teaching and skilful practice, Hippocrates became known to his contemporaries, such as Plato, as 'the famous physician', and to subsequent scholars not only as 'the father of medicine', but also as an eminent philosopher, historian, and writer. He travelled widely before dying in Thessaly in approximately 370 BC.

Hippocrates and his followers produced nearly sixty treatises on the causes and symptoms of disease and on the practice of medicine. The Hippocratic Corpus incorporates a variety of different textual styles and theoretical approaches, including: detailed accounts of specific types of disease, such as *Epidemics*, *Diseases of Women*, and *On the Sacred Disease* (epilepsy); manuals offering advice on clinical problems, including *The Book of Prognostics* and *On Regimen in Acute Diseases*; philosophical, but pragmatic, reflections on contemporary theories of disease, evident in both *On the Nature of Man* and *On Airs, Waters, and Places*; the epigrammatic *Aphorisms*, which became a standard educational text for medieval and Renaissance medical students; and the Hippocratic Oath, which has retained its legal and ethical significance into the modern period.

In Hippocratic medicine, health and disease, as well as character and personality, were thought to be determined by balance or imbalance in the four bodily humours: blood, phlegm, yellow bile, and black bile. An excess or depletion of one or more humours led to obstruction or dysfunction in the organs, leading to the signs and symptoms of disease. Diagnosis was made by taking a history and by thorough observation and examination of the patient's appearance, pulse, movement, and excretions. In general, treatment was gentle and expectant, allowing the natural healing power of the body (*vis medicatrix naturae*) to exert its effect, aided by careful attention to diet, exercise, sleep, and the environment, and only occasionally bolstered by more invasive therapies such as herbal remedies, massage, bloodletting, and purging.

The Corpus contains a number of references to breathing difficulties, for which the Hippocratic authors used a variety of overlapping terms: dyspnoea constituted a general and mild form of respiratory discomfort; orthopnoea was used to denote laboured breathing exacerbated by lying down and eased by sitting or standing; tachypnoea referred to rapid breathing; and the term 'asthma', sometimes appearing in the plural form as 'asthmas' (*asthmata*), described a discrete condition or set of conditions marked by relatively severe breathing difficulties. In *On the Nature of Bones*, for example, Hippocrates described the manner in which foreign bodies lodged in the lungs could impede 'both inhalation and exhalation...producing tachypnoea and dyspnoea. This situation results in diseases like asthma and dry phthisis.'[3]

Within this conceptual framework, asthma was regarded as the product of excess phlegm. In some phlegmatic patients, accumulations of phlegm in the brain caused convulsions or seizures, in which the 'patient loses his speech, and chokes, and foam issues by the mouth, the teeth are fixed, the hands are contracted, the eyes distorted, he becomes insensible, and in some cases the bowels are evacuated'. For Hippocrates, these classic manifestations of epilepsy were not expressions of a divine or sacred disease, as many believed, but the result of superfluous quantities of phlegm. However, if the phlegm flowed from the brain to the chest, other diseases eventually appeared:

> But should the defluxion make its way to the heart, the person is seized with palpitation and asthma, the chest becomes diseased, and some also have curvature of the spine. For when a defluxion of cold phlegm takes place on the lungs and heart, the blood is chilled, and the veins, being violently chilled, palpitate in the lungs and heart, and the heart palpitates, so that from this necessity asthma and orthopnoea supervene.[4]

It was perhaps for this reason that Hippocrates regarded convulsions and asthma as closely related conditions that were particularly common in infants. As Hippocrates explained in *On Airs, Waters, and Places*, these twin disorders were both more frequent in children living in cities that were exposed to hot winds, where the water was plentiful and salty, and the heads of the inhabitants were 'of a humid and pituitous constitution... [with] phlegm running down from the head'.[5] In addition to children being afflicted with asthma, the Hippocratic aphorisms suggest that the condition was also more common amongst the middle-aged and that attacks occurred most often during the autumn months. Significantly, given subsequent formulations of asthma as a relatively mild affliction, it is striking that the Hippocratic Corpus also acknowledged the potential severity of the condition: 'Such persons as become hump-backed from asthma or cough before puberty, die.'[6]

Hippocratic notions of asthma as a relatively distinct disorder, but one linked to other breathing difficulties, were perpetuated by other ancient medical authors, such as Erasistratus (*c*.315–240 BC), who founded a school of anatomy in Alexandria and whose work on respiration subsequently influenced Galen. During the first century AD, the Roman encyclopaedist Aulus Cornelius Celsus (25 BC–AD 50) also discussed asthma in his extensive popular writings on health and disease. Although his major work, *De medicina*, was written in Latin, the precise terminology employed by Celsus is instructive. Throughout most of the text, Celsus used Latin phrases (*spiritus difficultas, spiritus gravitas, tardum spiritum*, and *crebro spirare*) to describe the difficult or rapid breathing routinely associated with fevers, lung infections, obesity, and jaundice. In these conditions, laboured breathing generally constituted a poor prognostic sign. However, in one particular section, Celsus not only adopted the Greek words for certain breathing difficulties but also categorized the symptoms and the types of disease along Hippocratic lines, with particular reference to the noisy, gasping breathing characteristic of asthma:

> There is also in the region of the throat a malady which amongst the Greeks has different names according to its intensity. It consists altogether in a difficulty of breathing; when moderate and without any choking, it is called dyspnoea; when most severe, so that the patient cannot breathe without making a noise and gasping, asthma; but when in addition the patient can hardly draw in his breath unless with the neck outstretched, orthopnoea.[7]

Celsus' clinical description was also precise, providing a clear impression of the discomfort, debility, and expiratory wheeze caused by acute asthma attacks: 'on account of the narrow passage by which the breath escapes, it comes out with a whistle; there is pain in the chest and praecordia, at times even in the shoulder-blades, sometimes subsiding, then returning; to these there is added a slight cough.' Celsus' approach to treatment was probably more aggressive than that of the Hippocratic authors. He advised blood-letting as a standard remedy, supplemented by milk and clysters (or enemas) to loosen the bowels, hot foments, plasters, and emollients to ease chest movements, and diuretics, emetics, exercise, and massage to deplete the body and allow the patient to draw breath more easily. Herbal remedies included drinking hydromel (a mixture of honey and water) or mead containing hyssop or crushed caper roots, or sucking white nasturtium seeds mixed with honey. More particularly, Celsus also recommended either consuming the liver of a fox, dried and pounded and sprinkled into a cupful of wine, or eating the fresh, roasted lungs of the same animal.[8]

While Celsus was familiar and relatively comfortable with Greek terminology for breathing difficulties, other contemporary Roman authors deliberately distanced themselves from that tradition. In Book 23 of *The Natural History*, written in Latin, Pliny the Elder (AD 32–79), a renowned naval and military commander as well as author, did use the Greek term 'dyspnoea' to denote 'hardness of breathing', but elsewhere preferred the Latin terms *anhelitum*, *anhelationibus*, or *suspiriosis* to describe shortness of breath. For Pliny, popular remedies for difficulty breathing included oil of balsamum, rue combined with bitumen, pitched wines unless respiratory symptoms were accompanied by a fever, and the 'blood of wild horses taken in drink'.[9]

Pliny's contemporary, the Stoic philosopher Lucius Annaeus Seneca (4 BC–AD 65), was more dismissive of the learned practice of adopting Greek linguistic fashions. Born in Cordoba in Roman Spain, Seneca led a colourful life, but one that was tainted by chronic disease, including asthma, for which he spent several years in the drier, warmer climate of Egypt during his youth. Having trained in law, he became an elected official in the Roman treasury and a leading speaker in the Senate, before being banished to Corsica for eight years, supposedly for committing adultery with Julia Livilla, Caligula's sister. During his enforced exile Seneca continued to write, and when he returned to Rome in AD 49 he became Nero's tutor. Seneca retired from public life in AD 62, but, as a result of a conspiracy against Nero three years later in which he was implicated, he was compelled by the emperor to commit suicide.

During the last three years of his life, Seneca devoted his time and energy to writing, becoming one of the most influential philosophers in the Western Christian world. In the process, he produced perhaps the first clear personal account of what it was like to suffer from asthma, although he preferred not to use that term. In his fifty-fourth letter to Lucilius, a civil servant from Pompeii and the procurator of Sicily, Seneca not only provided a vivid description of the manner in which he 'gasped for breath' during an acute attack of asthma or dyspnoea, but also resisted the uncritical acceptance of Greek terminology for the condition:

> There's one particular ailment, though, for which I've always been singled out, so to speak. I see no reason to call it by its Greek name, difficulty in breathing being a perfectly good way of describing it. Its onslaught is of very brief duration—like a squall, it is generally over within the hour. One could hardly, after all, expect anyone to keep on drawing his last breath for long, could one? I have suffered every kind of unpleasant or dangerous physical complaint, but none is worse than this. Not surprising, for anything else is just an illness, while this is gasping out your life-breath. That is why doctors call it a "rehearsal for death", since eventually the breath does what it has often been trying to do.[10]

In a later letter, Seneca also emphasized the value of adopting a stoical philosophical mentality in order to endure the distress of illness, in this instance chronic catarrh, from which Seneca, like Lucilius, suffered along with asthma. In addition to acknowledging the importance of a suitable Hippocratic regimen of appropriate levels of exercise, purposeful activity, and a healthy diet, Seneca was also keen to prescribe, like many other ancient authors, 'a remedy not just for this ailment but for your life as a whole'. In order to combat 'the fear of death, the physical pain, and the interruption to our pleasures' that accompany every illness, Seneca proposed philosophy and friendship to improve mental health, diversions and distractions to banish negative preoccupations with pain, and a determination to fight, rather than succumb to, illness and adversity.[11]

Although Seneca and Pliny attempted to resist the long-established dominance of Greek disease terminology, most classical medical authorities, whether writing in Greek or Latin, began routinely to adopt the words 'asthma', 'orthopnoea', and 'dyspnoea' for varying degrees and manifestations of respiratory distress. In the first century AD, for example, both Rufus (AD 30–100) in *Quaestiones Medicinales*, and Dioscorides (*c.* AD 40–90) in his extensive encyclopaedia of herbal remedies *De Materia Medica*, referred to the features and treatment of asthma. According to Dioscorides, a wide variety of aromatic plant extracts were effective against asthma, orthopnoea, and other forms of breathing difficulties: the juice of the balsam tree given with milk; the sap from Arabic gum trees; perfumes such as cyphi; the fragrant root of horse elder; bitter almond oil; the sap of a myrrh tree taken in pill form; a linctus containing pitch pine; bitumen for obstinate coughs and asthma; the leaves of the weeping cypress, bruised and taken with wine; the juice of a raw quince; figs boiled with hyssop and taken as a drink; and sweet bay or laurel in a linctus with honey or raisin wine.[12]

At much the same time, Aretaeus of Cappadocia (*c.* AD 50–150) produced one of the most expansive ancient clinical accounts of asthma in *On the Causes and Symptoms of Chronic Disease*. Writing in Ionic Greek and largely following the Hippocratic method, Aretaeus regarded health and disease as the product of balance or imbalance between the four humours and 'pneuma', a specific form of air or spirit. The maintenance of health required

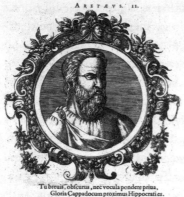

Tu breuis, obscurus, nec vocula pondere priua,
Gloria Cappadocum proximus Hippocrati es.
Goupylusà tineis feruar, te Crassus honorus
Induit Ausonia veste: legére diu.

2. Aretaeus, c. AD 50–150.
(*Wellcome Library, London*)

in particular the unimpeded flow of pneuma through the blood vessels, a process that could be facilitated by bleeding, purgatives, and the administration of narcotics.

Aretaeus began his description of asthma in familiar Homeric style.

> If from running, gymnastic exercise, or any other work, the breathing becomes difficult, it is called *Asthma*; and the disease *Orthopnoea* is also called Asthma, for in the paroxysms the patients also pant for breath. The disease is called *Orthopnoea*, because it is only when in an erect position that they breathe freely; for when reclined there is a sense of suffocation.

Locating the disease distinctly in the lungs, Aretaeus attributed asthma to 'a coldness and humidity of the spirit (*Pneuma*); but the *materiel* is a thick and viscid humour'. While women were more likely to suffer from asthma, because 'they are humid and cold', men were likely to die more speedily from the condition. Recovery could be anticipated, however, in those whose lungs were heated 'in the exercise of their trade, from being wrapped in wool, such as the workers in gypsum, or braziers, or black-smiths, or the heaters of baths'.[13]

According to Aretaeus, the symptoms of a nascent attack of asthma included heaviness in the chest, tiredness, and difficulty breathing at work or on exertion, a cough, flatulence, and rest-lessness, a slight fever at night, and a 'nose sharp and ready for respiration'. For those patients who escaped a 'fatal termina-tion', the symptoms might recede, but 'traces of the affection' were evident even in remission. If the patient's condition deteri-orated, however, the symptoms and signs became more florid, with the risk of death:

> But if the evil gradually get worse, the cheeks are ruddy; eyes protruberant, as if from strangulation; a *râle* during the waking state, but the evil much worse in sleep; voice liquid and without resonance; a desire of much and of cold air; they eagerly go into the open air, since no house sufficeth for their respiration; they breathe standing, as if desiring to draw in all the air which they possibly can inhale; and, in their want of air, they also open the mouth as if thus to enjoy the more of it; pale in the countenance, except the cheeks, which are ruddy; sweat about the forehead and clavicles; cough incessant and laborious; expectoration small, thin, cold, resembling the efflorescence of foam; neck swells with the inflation of the breath (*pneuma*); the praecordia retracted; pulse small, dense, compressed; legs slender: and if these symptoms increase, they sometimes produce suffocation, after the form of epilepsy.[14]

In the following chapter, Aretaeus also described a particularly malignant form of asthma, referred to as 'pneumodes', in which 'dyspnoea, cough, insomnolency, and heat are common symp-toms, as also loss of appetite and general emaciation', and from which patients usually died within a year. Although the precise relationship between this condition and other manifestations of asthma is unclear, Aretaeus' description of the pathology of the condition is interesting, since it betrays a close familiarity with morbid anatomy, possibly obtained from post-mortem dissections. In patients with this condition, coughing either failed to result in expectoration or produced only 'a small, white, round substance, resembling a hailstone'. While the lungs were free from suppuration, they were found to be filled with 'compacted humours'.[15]

Aretaeus' account of asthma demonstrates the clinical acumen, as well as the nosological or diagnostic flexibility, of many ancient physicians. Similar characteristics are also evident in the work of Aretaeus' more famous contemporary Galen (c. AD 129–210). Born in Pergamum in AD 129, Galen served as an attendant in a local healing temple before travelling to study in Smyrna, Corinth, and Alexandria. After a further period as a physician in Pergamum, in AD 162 he moved to Rome, where he continued to teach and practise medicine and to compose medical treatises. Apart from spending some time in his native city between AD 166 and 169, Galen remained in Rome, where he treated many elite Roman dignitaries before he died in approximately AD 210.

Galen was a prolific writer, whose works, composed originally in Greek but regularly translated into Syriac, Arabic, and Latin during the medieval period, became influential throughout the Western, Middle Eastern, and Eastern worlds. Clearly informed by his education in philosophy, by his close knowledge of the Hippocratic Corpus, and by his own anatomical experiments, Galen's major medical works include *On the Natural Faculties*, *On the Affected Parts*, *On the Doctrines of Hippocrates and Plato*, *On the Usefulness of the Parts of the Body*, *On Prognosis*, and,

more pertinently in the present context, a treatise on breathing difficulties, *De difficultate respirationis.* Throughout these writings, Galen espoused a model of health and disease that drew
not only on Hippocrates but also on Aristotle. In essence, Galen
regarded disease as the result of imbalances in the four funda-
mental qualities: hot, cold, wet, and dry. Critically, since certain
environments or substances could cause disease by disturbing
what was deemed to be a healthy, natural balance, alteration of
environmental circumstances or the administration of extracts
from plants, animals, and minerals could also be used for therapeutic purposes. While Galen's approach to the classification
and causes of disease was thus essentially Hippocratic, his remedies were more aggressive and included a far greater range of
pharmacological preparations as well as blood-letting.

Galen was particularly interested in the physiology of respiration, performing a series of experiments, largely on pigs, to
demonstrate the role of the diaphragm and intercostal muscles in
breathing. Drawing on, and often contesting, the earlier physiological works of Erasistratus, Galen, like Aretaeus, believed in
the existence and importance of pneuma, a vital principle that
was inhaled during respiration and was distributed through
the body by the circulatory system. Significantly, in addition to
investigating normal respiration, Galen also explored the clinical features of breathing difficulties. He emphasized the importance of observing the movement of the chest wall in patients
suffering from dyspnoea, since muscle weaknesses and injury
were often responsible for breathing difficulties.[16]

More particularly, Galen included almost seventy references
to asthma, or derivatives of that word, in his medical writings,
some in connection with his commentaries on the Hippocratic
aphorisms and others in relation to his own formulation of

breathing difficulties. As Armelle Debru has suggested in her expansive study of Galen's theories of respiration, Galen used the term 'asthma' in a number of ways: in a popular, Homeric sense to describe panting or breathlessness triggered by physical exertion; as a general form of dyspnoea caused by a broad range of acute, sometimes febrile, illnesses; and as a chronic respiratory disorder without fever. Galen did differentiate in some ways between different conditions: while dyspnoea comprised merely disordered breathing, asthma was marked more particularly by rapid, as well as laboured, breathing. However, in parallel with other classical authors, Galen continued to use the term 'asthma' in rather imprecise ways without a fixed meaning.[17]

According to Galen, the symptoms of asthma were caused primarily by obstruction in the lungs. In On the Affected Parts, which constitutes a discussion of diseases arranged according to the principal organ involved, Galen suggested that 'if the breathing is rough and noisy it indicates that a large amount of thick and sticky humors in the bronchial tubes of the lungs has accumulated and become annoying because it is difficult to expectorate'. Equally, he contrasted the often fatal outcome in patients with empyema with the favourable prognosis in asthma in similar terms: 'in asthmatic affections, when sticky and thick humours fill up the lungs, the patients remain strong and vigorous.'[18] Consequently, Galenic treatment involved adopting a suitable lifestyle and taking appropriate medication aimed at restoring the balance of the elements and reducing the accretion of humours in the lungs.

In many ways, Galen epitomizes classical approaches to asthma. The term itself had become an accepted element of the medical vocabulary, and, although the boundaries between asthma and other respiratory conditions were not clearly drawn, there were suggestions that asthma was beginning to constitute a distinct chronic condition with its own characteristic constellation of symptoms: breathlessness; whistling exhalation; cough; difficulty breathing lying down; and distress. Many other authors in antiquity, including Aretaeus, Celsus, Seneca, and Pliny, promoted similar accounts of asthma and recommended a wide range of specific herbal treatments or generic advice concerning diet and exercise, but few of their works were cited by subsequent writers until their rediscovery during the Renaissance. It was almost exclusively the works of Galen, and partly through Galen those of Hippocrates, that were transmitted to provide a template for the development of Islamic medicine and to inspire medieval commentators on asthma.

Medieval treatises

The history of asthma, like the history of disease in general, in many ways reflects the cultural and political history of the world. After the collapse of the Graeco-Roman empire and the expansion of Arabia into Syria, Egypt, and Iraq during the sixth and seventh centuries, classical medicine declined: manuscripts were burned or lost; medicine retreated into the monasteries; and it was left to Byzantine, Islamic, and Jewish scholars to refine and transmit ancient knowledge of asthma and other conditions. Only the careful translation of Hippocratic and Galenic texts into Syriac, Arabic, Hebrew, and eventually Latin served to preserve classical accounts of asthma.

The move to safeguard and promulgate the works of Galen and Hippocrates in particular had been initiated in the early Byzantine period by medical authors such as Oribasius (c.320–400). Born in Pergamum, Oribasius became physician to the

Roman emperor Julian and a magistrate in Constantinople. He was essentially a prodigious encyclopaedist, whose monumental *Collectiones Medicae*, written in Greek, contains excerpts from many of the classical Greek and Roman physicians and became a standard text for medical students. The compendium of medical knowledge compiled by Oribasius incorporates extracts from, and commentaries on, much of Galen's work, including some of his lost writings on respiration, particularly *On the Movement of the Lungs and Thorax* and *On the Cause of Respiration*, thereby helping to establish Galen's continuing influence during the following centuries.[19]

Authoritative commentaries on ancient medical authors were also compiled by Stephanus of Athens in the sixth or seventh century. Like the works of Oribasius, Stephanus' published commentaries on the Hippocratic aphorisms and on *The Book of Prognostics* were intended primarily to serve as educational tools and were derived from a course of lectures delivered to medical students in Alexandria. In Stephanus' writings, the succinct style of the Hippocratic authors was expanded and developed to produce an intricate picture of health and disease that merged clinical knowledge of the body with contemporary beliefs about humoral balance and environmental conditions. In Section III, Aphorism 22, for example, Hippocrates suggested that a number of diseases, including asthma, were more common in autumn, partly, according to Stephanus, because the colder weather thickened the bilious humour that had accumulated during the summer. For Stephanus, Hippocrates was using the term 'asthma' in two ways in this section: as a general term for difficult breathing, caused, for example, by a quinsy or sore throat; or in a more specific sense to denote the obstruction of vessels in the lungs, 'thus causing difficult breathing, i.e. asthma'.[20]

In his discussion of later aphorisms, Stephanus explored more concisely what Hippocrates meant by asthma and its causes:

> We know already what asthma is: quick and frequent breathing. And how do we explain the asthma? There is an inward pressure on the vertebrae at the occiput, it presses on the esophagus, which presses on the larynx and thus narrows the air passage, so that there is quick and frequent breathing, called asthma by Hippocrates.[21]

Stephanus similarly extended Hippocrates' discussion of the prevalence of asthma in middle age. Stephanus' explanation for the clinical appearance of asthma later in life effectively integrated understandings of temperament, life cycle, and season into a complex philosophy of medicine and living that demonstrated the continued authority of humoral models of disease.

> Middle age is characterized by an irregular temperament, and by this irregularity of temperament the natural faculties are weakened, in consequence of which various and manifold diseases are produced in this group; in the same way autumn with its irregular temperament produces various and manifold bad humors, which naturally cause various and manifold diseases owing to the weakening of the faculties, since irregularity of any kind weakens the faculties and upsets the constitution...middle age is analogous to autumn, the prime of life to summer; and because of this analogy, just as autumn is the cause of many various diseases, so there are many various diseases which middle age tends to produce.
>
> These people are prone to asthma. We have heard more than once what asthma is: heavy and very fast breathing. The asthma is easily explained by the irregularity of the temperament. Phlegm is produced by weakening of the faculties and failure to digest the food; this phlegm flows to the pharynx, the larynx, and the trachea, thus the air is prevented from passing, and this causes asthma.[22]

As the works of many ancient and medieval medical writers suggest, the symptoms of asthma occurred either alone or in conjunction with other conditions. One of the most intriguing connections suggested in medieval treatises is contained in the work of the prominent Islamic physician Abū Bakr Muḥammad ibn Zakarīyā' al-Rāzī (865–c.925), known in medieval Europe as Rhazes. Born in Iran, al-Rāzī completed his medical education in Baghdad before practising medicine and directing hospitals first in his home town of Rayy and subsequently in Baghdad. He wrote extensively, not only shaping the development of medicine but also contributing widely to the study of philosophy, alchemy, mathematics, theology, and music. Although some of his writings constituted compilations of Greek, Syrian, Indian, and Arabic medical knowledge, he was an independent and highly critical thinker who challenged established medical and religious authorities. From a medical perspective, he questioned the interpretations of Galen on occasions and aligned himself more directly with Hippocratic approaches to the observation, diagnosis, and treatment of disease.

Two particular accounts of respiratory disease by al-Rāzī are instructive. In one of the surviving volumes of his *al-Kitāb al-Ḥāwī fī ṭibb*, known as *The Comprehensive Book on Medicine*, al-Rāzī discussed a patient who was suffering from severe attacks of *coryza*, or runny nose. Significantly, the symptoms often moved to the chest: 'Even the slighter form of it used to remain with the sufferer a month or more and to descend to the chest, causing coughing and expectoration.'[23] In a letter advising a friend how to prevent or treat similar symptoms provoked specifically by exposure to pollinating flowers during spring, al-Rāzī provided what some historical commentators have suggested was the first clinical account of hay fever or allergic rhinitis. Al-Rāzī may also have recognized a link between a running nose, itching, and sneezing, on the one hand, and asthmatic symptoms, on the other hand: he noted, for example, that nasal symptoms in such cases were often accompanied by 'coughing, tightness of breath and breathlessness'. Treatment included not only avoiding perfumed plants and applying various herbal remedies, but also adopting strategies to improve breathing, such as inhalations to loosen mucus in the lungs, and advice on the best position for sleeping.[24]

Evidence that al-Rāzī was describing a form of asthma triggered by exposure to pollen comes from the work of later medical writers whose treatises regularly included references to Arabic authors, as well as to the Greek medical authority of Hippocrates and Galen. In the present context, it is particularly significant that subsequent treatises on asthma not only cited and analysed al-Rāzī's philosophy of medicine, such as his aphorisms, but also substantiated his specific approach to the treatment of asthma, most notably his use of hart's tongue and fig juice to expel phlegm and ease breathing. It may well be, therefore, that al-Rāzī's discussion of *coryza* and breathlessness induced by contact with flowering plants constituted an early recognition of what later became an established association between hay fever and asthma.[25]

Al-Rāzī's contemporaries also considered the symptoms and clinical signs of asthma in their medical treatises. In his *Breviary*, which was written in the late ninth or tenth century in Arabic and translated into Latin in the twelfth century, Yuhanna ibn Sarabyoun (870–930), referred to in Latin editions as Johannes Filius Serapionis, explained the presentation of asthma, and its overlap with other conditions, in typical ancient terms. Asthmatic breathing difficulties, he argued, were caused by the accumulation of 'thick and phlegmatic humor' in the lungs, not only leading patients to fear that they would 'suffocate' during an attack but also forcing them to sit upright, as in earlier Greek descriptions of orthopnoea, in an attempt to alleviate respiratory distress: 'Therefore, they straighten their chest and neck until they are able to breathe. This is why this disease is called "straightness of breathing" (*directio anhelitus*), because someone with this disease is unable to breathe unless sitting up.'[26]

Approximately one century later, perhaps the most influential medieval medical author, Ibn Sīnā (980–1037), more usually known in the West as Avicenna, included an extensive account of asthma in his *Kitāb al-Qānūn fī al-ṭibb* or *Canon of Medicine*. Ibn Sīnā was born in Afshana, near Bukhara in Uzbekistan, and during an itinerant life produced nearly 300 works on mathematics, law, theology, philosophy, and medicine. Comprising five books, which focused in turn on the general principles of medicine, simple remedies, anatomically specific diseases (including diseases of the lungs and chest), systemic conditions, and the medicinal use of compound drugs, Ibn Sīnā's *Canon* was translated into Latin by Gerard of Cremona (1114–87) in the late twelfth century and became a standard educational text for medical students in Italy during the Renaissance and early modern period.

According to Ibn Sīnā, asthma was a chronic disease in which patients often suffered 'acute paroxysms with similarity to the paroxysms of epilepsy and spasm'. The flow of thick humours from the head to the lungs produced a situation in which 'the patient finds no escape from rapid panting, like the labored panting of one who is being choked or rushed'. Treatment reflected ancient and medieval preoccupations with regimen and incorporated a combination of approaches: purging, vomiting, and blood-letting; voice exercises; foods such as the 'fats of hares and deer and gazelles and the penises of foxes and above all their lungs'; arsenic, in the form of pills with pine resin, given in a drink with honey water, or administered by inhalation; and sulphur, taken either in water with soft-boiled eggs or by inhalation.[27]

While the works of al-Rāzī and Ibn Sīnā were certainly influential, it was the Jewish scholar Rabbi Moses ben Maimon Maimonides (1138–1204) who produced probably the first medical treatise devoted entirely to asthma. Maimonides was born in Córdoba in Spain in 1138. He gained fame as a doctor and philosopher, becoming both court physician under Saladin the Great in Cairo and the leader of the Jewish community in Egypt. His publications, which were written in Arabic but often translated into Hebrew, included commentaries on the works of Galen and Hippocrates, medical texts on specific conditions such as asthma, sexual intercourse, poisons, and fits, and a wide range of influential theological and philosophical commentaries. Maimonides died in Palestine in 1204.

Maimonides's treatise on asthma constitutes a lucid and well-organized account of contemporary knowledge of the condition. It was translated at least three times into Hebrew during the fourteenth century and twice into Latin in the fourteenth and fifteenth centuries, but it was not until recently that an English version was available. The medical advice imparted is similar in content and approach to that offered by Maimonides's *On the Regimen of Health* (1198), which provided a broad introduction to the manner in which careful attention to what were generally known as the six 'non-naturals' (air, food and drink, movement and rest, emotions, sleep, and excretion) and to the frequency of sexual intercourse could effectively preserve or restore health. In repeating much of this general advice in the treatise on asthma, Maimonides was reinforcing and disseminating an ancient and medieval commitment to the importance of a moderate lifestyle in maintaining humoral balance and health.

The treatise on asthma was written by Maimonides in response to a patient's request for advice; it therefore constitutes not only a dissertation on asthma but also a regimen for health adapted to the patient's individual needs. According to Maimonides, chronic asthma was not uncommon, and the causes were well known to medieval physicians. Contemporary understandings of the disease drew heavily on Hippocratic formulations of humoral excess:

> the cause of this asthma [from which he suffers] is a defluxion that descends from the brain at certain times [of the year], but mostly in winter. And I know that the orthopnoea and distress do not cease through the night for days on end, according to the length or brevity of the attack, until the defluxion decreases and until that [fluid] which has reached the lungs has been cocted [modified by the body to aid elimination] so that the latter have become clean.[28]

The patient's asthma in this instance was exacerbated by hot foods and by wearing a turban, since they increased heat in the brain, and was eased by a move to Cairo, where the air was 'lighter and calmer'. Accordingly, Maimonides set out a comprehensive range of instructions for alleviating asthma that aimed to restore humoral balance and reduce the accumulation of phlegm by paying close attention, in the first instance, to the non-naturals and to sexual intercourse. While he acknowledged, like Ibn Sīnā, that cure was unlikely in most chronic diseases of this nature, Maimonides nevertheless suggested that adherence to 'a good regimen ... necessarily prolongs the interval between the cycles and diminishes the occurrences [of attacks] in a cycle, alleviates the suffering and pain which they cause, and makes it easier to bear them'.[29]

Diet was crucial to the medieval management of chronic asthma. The physician's intention was to ensure that 'all the veins and passages are open and clean and free from obstructions and constriction so that the pneumas and humors stream through them [freely] and the superfluities are expelled'.[30] To achieve this, Maimonides recommended a wide range of foods, many of which had been recognized as beneficial for asthmatics by ancient commentators: pickled fish with a 'purgative and attenuating effect'; the meat, and especially lungs, of foxes, identified as therapeutic many centuries earlier by Celsus; the fat of rabbits; a variety of vegetables; raisins, quinces, dried figs, and nuts to loosen and thin the humours; moderate amounts of wine, or various non-alcoholic alternatives for Muslims, taken some time after a meal in order to expel 'the superfluities by means of perspiration and urine'; and a selection of broths or gruels, particularly those made from barley, which had been recommended by Hippocrates, Galen, Aristotle, and Pliny for its nourishing, cleansing, and cooling properties.

Equally importantly, Maimonides advised avoiding or restricting the consumption of those foods that produced 'thick or sticky humors' or were 'rich in superfluities'. Foods that increased the accumulation of phlegm and exacerbated asthma included: milk and cheese, which 'fill the head and harm the brain'; the meat of geese and ducks, which 'contain many corrupt humours'; bread made from 'thoroughly sifted' flour; juicy fresh fruits, such as melon, peach, apricot, mulberry, cucumber, dates, and grapes, which were thought to cause flatulence; any hot and dry ingredients, such as spices, which made the 'fatty humors sticky and thicken and coagulate those humors which have no fatness'; and excess consumption of wine, 'especially [to the point of] drunkenness'.[31]

Having briefly noted the importance of avoiding cold, moist air, Maimonides also recognized the impact of emotions on asthma, and indeed on health generally. In Chapter Eight of the treatise, he noted that sadness, fear, worry, and distress could reduce appetite, weaken the lungs, and deplete energy; if a poor state of mind persisted, illness and death could result. Conversely, much as Seneca had suggested in his letters to Lucilius in the first century AD, 'joy and pleasure have an effect opposite to all these things because of the dilation of the soul and the movement of the blood and pneuma to the outside of the body so that the functions of the organs seem to be at their very best'. However, Maimonides was aware that the treatment of emotional distress, and the consequent physical symptoms, did not fall within the province of medicine; suffering was to be alleviated by an ethical philosophy that served to subdue passions and to reduce the transitory but harmful influences of 'mere anger or pleasure'.[32]

Humoral imbalances were also to be corrected by preventing the retention of urine or faeces, and by encouraging the removal of superfluous humours with appropriate dietary modifications, supplemented by emetics and enemas only if necessary. In addition, patients with asthma were advised to sleep as little as possible, especially during an attack or after a meal, since sleep filled 'the brain with vapors', and to avoid bathing in cold water, which closed the body's pores and facilitated the accumulation of phlegm. Maimonides also advised his readers, particularly the elderly, to avoid excessive sexual intercourse, which depleted the body of 'vital fluids and innate heat', and to massage the chest or take exercise only between asthmatic attacks.[33]

As Maimonides admitted throughout his discussion of the role of the non-naturals in maintaining or restoring health, many of these generic treatments for chronic disease were derived from Galen's recommendations, although Maimonides carefully selected and modified those Galenic preparations that were, in his experience, the most effective and the most suitable for his patients. For example, he particularly recommended enemas of linseed or fenugreek, both combined with olive oil, chicken fat, and beet juice, to facilitate 'evacuation of the stools in a smooth way without causing irritation or harm'. In some instances, Maimonides also experimented with certain preparations intended to improve digestion and remove phlegm: 'I experimented upon myself and took one ounce of white sugar pulverized with half a *dirham* of anise in the wintertime; in the summertime I drank it with a little lemon juice every third or fourth day...I found that it purifies the stomach from phlegm and cleanses it well.'[34]

Having established a suitable regimen for asthmatic patients, Maimonides explored the prescription of more specific remedies. Asthma was notoriously difficult to cure: rubefacients or blistering drugs tended to weaken the brain by heating it, while cooling drugs served to coagulate the humours and obstruct the lungs. For this reason, according to Maimonides, patients should entrust themselves only to experienced doctors who were capable of preparing suitable compounds and observing their clinical effects, rather than resorting to the advice of mere empiricists. In principle, if the general regimen was faithfully adhered to, Maimonides hoped that drugs would be necessary only 'once a year in the springtime'.[35]

Acute attacks were to be treated along Galenic lines. Ideally, patients were to start with a dilute preparation of any remedy and to alternate treatments to achieve maximum effect. In mild attacks, a combination of sugar beverages, soup made from young chickens, and a linctus was often sufficient to cleanse the lungs and reduce breathlessness. In more severe attacks, more aggressive treatments were necessary: decoctions, purgatives, enemas, and fumigations were required to remove superfluous humours, strengthen the brain, prevent the flow of humours to the lungs, and ease expectoration. In each case, Maimonides provided his readers with simple recipes to facilitate the preparation of complex mixtures of flowering plants, fruits, animal extracts, and liquids.

Certain medieval treatments are particularly significant within the longer history of asthma. While later authors debated the merits of narcotics in the treatment of asthma attacks, Maimonides himself recommended opium syrup, prepared from 'fresh, ripe white poppy', since it was thought to prevent defluxions, aid sleep, and thicken the phlegm, thereby easing expectoration. In addition, Maimonides stressed the importance of inhalations and fumigations, which became one of the foundations of Marcel Proust's desperate attempts to alleviate his asthma in the early twentieth century. In particular, Maimonides described the manner in which aloe or a mixture of arsenic, long birthwort, and ox fat, for example, should be 'cast into a fire so that its vapor enters the nostrils and the mouth'.[36]

Concluding with reflections on the regimens of health and the philosophies of medicine promoted by Hippocrates, Galen, al-Rāzī, and Ibn Sīnā, Maimonides's treatise offers an intimate account of late-medieval approaches to asthma and other chronic diseases. Respectful of his patient's status and individual needs and sensitive to the distress caused by asthma, Maimonides carefully explored the range of therapeutic options available to medieval doctors and their patients. It is important to stress that, while Maimonides's approach to the causes of asthma and his prescriptions for its prevention and treatment rested heavily on ancient formulations of disease, he was not merely passively reciting classical views: his therapeutic approach also incorporated the results of his own clinical experience, observations, and preferences.

Like the work of many Byzantine, Islamic, and Jewish scholars in the medieval period, the writings of al-Rāzī, Ibn Sīnā, and Maimonides did much not only to synthesize and preserve the views of ancient authors on asthma until European interest in classical medicine was reignited during the Renaissance, but also to promote interest in a wider range of pharmacological remedies, many of which were unknown to the Greeks. The medieval period was, therefore, no dark age. Often through Latin translations, the works of these Middle Eastern scholars were well known to, and widely cited by, medical students and physicians at the emerging medical schools in Salerno, Bologna, and Montpellier. Greek, Latin, Syriac, Arabic, and Hebrew treatises produced between the seventh and twelfth centuries provided the theoretical and clinical basis from which late-medieval and early Renaissance scholars in Italy and France, such as Taddeo Alderotti (c.1215–95), William of Brescia (c.1250–1326), and Bernard of Gordon (c.1258–1330), began to compose their own formulations of the clinical manifestations and treatment of asthma.[37]

Eastern traditions

Although the term 'asthma' itself was conceived by a Greek literary imagination and nurtured by Islamic and Jewish scholars, shortness of breath and related breathing difficulties were also recognized and treated by medical practitioners in other ancient cultures. Towards the end of his treatise on asthma, Maimonides cited examples not only from classical Greek and Roman medicine but also significantly from Egyptian medical theories and procedures with which he had become closely acquainted during his long career in Cairo. There remains some dispute as to whether ancient Egyptian medicine identified a form of breathing difficulty directly comparable with asthma. The Ebers papyrus, discovered in a tomb at Thebes in 1862 and named after the German professor Georg Ebers, who purchased the papyrus in 1873, is one of the oldest extant records of medical practice. Compiled in approximately 1550 BC but representing medical knowledge stretching back a further millennium or so, the papyrus details a series of recipes for a diverse range of medical, ophthalmological, and surgical conditions. Believing disease to be the product of maleficent humours, such as phlegm, the Egyptians prescribed a wide range of chemical formulations, as well as prayers and incantations, to remove harmful matter and restore health.

According to one of the earliest English translations of the Ebers papyrus by Ebbell in 1937, Egyptian doctors recognized and treated asthma. Ebbell suggests that the Egyptians described only two forms of respiratory symptom, cough and asthma, and that they were therefore unable to differentiate between many lung diseases. While Ebbell's specific interpretation has been challenged by other translators, the papyrus certainly appears to list remedies to remove phlegm, alleviate catarrh, *coryza*, and coughs, and to ease breathing. Significantly, Egyptian treatments for respiratory conditions included not only the oral consumption of a variety of concocted vegetable, mineral, and animal products but also the delivery of active substances directly to the lungs by inhalation, which came to play such a significant part in the treatment of asthma in many later cultures:

> Thou shalt fetch 7 stones and heat them by the fire, thou shalt take one thereof and place (a little) of these remedies on it and cover it with a new vessel whose bottom is perforated and place a stalk of a reed in this hole; thou shalt put thy mouth to this stalk, so that thou inhalest the smoke of it. Likewise with all stones. Thereafter thou shalt eat something fat, of fat meat or oil.[38]

In many ways, Egyptian medicine provided the theoretical and practical basis for Graeco-Roman approaches to disease. Egyptian medical theories included an emphasis on humours, such as phlegm (śtt in Egyptian hieratic texts), and many of the medicinal plants recommended in the papyri were also subsequently listed by Dioscorides. Egyptian models of disease and approaches to treatment also continued to influence medieval authors, such as Maimonides and al-Rāzī. In addition to Maimonides's explicit acknowledgement of Egyptian medical philosophies in his treatise on asthma, certain causal connections evident in the papyri were explored, in symptomatic terms, in al-Rāzī's work. According to the Ebers papyrus, for example, śtt denoted not only phlegm but also rheumatic pains; similarly, al-Rāzī made a connection between *coryza* and subsequent 'pain in the articulations' caused by the flow of residue to the joints.[39]

Egyptian medicine was not the only ancient cultural tradition beyond Greece and Rome to recognize and treat breathing difficulties. Strongly shaped by Daoist and Buddhist conceptions of the cosmos, traditional Chinese medicine, like much Egyptian and Greek medicine, was built on the related notions of balance and flow. In the earliest medical writings from China, health and disease were understood in terms of the relative proportions of the polar opposites, yin and yang, and the flow of Qi (or *ch'i*, variably translated as wind or energy), which corresponded in some ways to the ancient Greek concept of pneuma. Although Chinese medicine was probably not formalized in written texts until the Han dynasty (between 206 BC and AD 220), it was based on the oral traditions of legendary rulers, such as Shen Nung, also known as the Divine Farmer or the Fire Emperor, and the Yellow Emperor Huang Di, who both held power and practised medicine during the third millennium BC.

According to some historians of Chinese medicine, it was Shen Nung who compiled the first Chinese *materia medica* or pharmacopoeia (*Pen-Ts'ao*), in which he described the therapeutic application of various plants. Among the substances recommended in the *Pen-Ts'ao* was *ma huang* or ephedra, a native plant of Asia and America that produces edible berries. Within the Chinese medical tradition, drinks prepared from the bitter-tasting stems of *ma huang* were regularly prescribed by doctors for a variety of respiratory conditions including 'plant fever, cough and eructations'.[40] Over subsequent centuries, *ma huang* not only became a standard remedy for shortness of breath within Chinese medicine but, as will become apparent, also furnished Western medicine with new treatments for asthma and hay fever.[41]

Respiratory symptoms were also discussed in the *Classic of Internal Medicine*, or *Nei Ching*, traditionally ascribed to Huang Di. Composed in the form of a dialogue between the emperor and his physician, Ch'i Po, the *Classic* provides clear details of the philosophy and practice of ancient Chinese medicine, according to which diagnoses were made particularly by examining the pulse, and treatment included acupuncture, moxibustion (a technique that involved burning herbs at selected sites on the surface of the body), massage, dietary changes, and spiritual guidance. In the final chapter of the *Classic*, which comprises a treatise on 'rebellion and harmony', the two men discuss the causes of noisy, troubled breathing:

> The Yellow Emperor said: 'Man is afflicted when he cannot rest and when his breathing has a sound (is noisy)—or when he cannot rest and his breathing is without any sound. He may rise and rest (his habits of life may be) as of old and his breathing is noisy; he may have his rest and his exercise and his breathing is troubled (wheezing, panting); or he may not be able to rest and be unable to walk about and his breathing is troubled. There are those who do not get a rest and those who rest and yet have troubled breathing. Is all this caused by the viscera? I desire to hear about their causes.'
>
> Ch'i Po answered: 'Those who do not rest and breathing is noisy have disorders in the region of Yang Ming (the "sunlight"). The Yang of the foot in descending causes the present disturbance and in ascending it causes the breathing to be noisy.'[42]

Published in the third century AD, Zhang Zhong Jing's *Essential Prescriptions of the Golden Chest* included discussions of both breathlessness or panting (*chuan*) and wheezing (*xiao*). Some centuries later, these symptoms were combined by Zhu Dan Xi (1281–1348) to produce the term *xiao chuan*, or 哮 喘. Although subsequent medical texts sometimes differentiated between the two conditions, many Chinese authorities came to regard *xiao chuan* as broadly equivalent to the Western term 'asthma'.[43] Ancient Chinese interpretations of breathing difficulties in terms of imbalances in yin and yang and obstruction to the flow of Qi by phlegm in the airways, as well as the central role of *ma huang* in restoring respiratory health, persisted. In Chinese medication charts from the fourteenth century, *xiao chuan* or

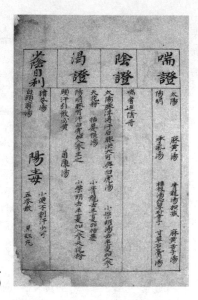

3. Chinese medication chart, 1341.
(*Wellcome Library, London*)

asthma occurred in different forms and was remedied with distinct herbal preparations: Greater Yang asthma was treated with ephedra or Variant Blue-Green Dragon decoction; patients with Yang Brightness asthma were prescribed Qi Supporting Decoction or liquorice and gypsum decoction; and Yin syndrome asthma was treated with Yin Returning elixir.

Chinese medical theories and practices influenced the development of medicine elsewhere in the Eastern world, particularly in Japan and Korea, where asthma was also recognized from antiquity. The 'Chinese method' of medicine, known in Japanese as *kanpō*, was introduced into Japan in the sixth century. Although infectious diseases such as smallpox, measles, and influenza dominated the pattern of disease and mortality in pre-modern Japan, asthma (*zensoku*) was referred to in medical texts and encyclopaedias written between AD 700 and 1600. In the twelfth and thirteenth centuries, the Japanese poet and calligrapher Fujiwara no Teika (1162–1241), who had a precarious relationship with Emperor Go-Toba and who supposedly fathered twenty-seven children, was reputed to have suffered from repeated bouts of asthma, bronchitis, and rheumatism that made him a semi-invalid.[44]

Korea was similarly afflicted by plagues during antiquity and the pre-modern period. However, as in the case of Japan, chronic respiratory diseases such as asthma also regularly appeared in Korean medical texts such as the *Hyang-yak kugup pang* (*Emergency Remedies of Folk Medicine*) compiled in 1236, the *Hyangyak chipsong pang* (*Compilation of Native Korean Prescriptions*) from 1433, and the *Tongui pogam* (*Exemplar of Korean Medicine*), written by the Daoist philosopher Ho Chun in 1610 in response to the decimation of the Korean population that occurred during the Hideyoshi Invasion between 1592 and 1598. Discussed largely in the context of 'coughing', asthma was divided into various forms and was thought to be triggered by 'excess eating, fear, and shock'. These texts remained influential, not only in Korea but also in China and Japan, well into the eighteenth century.[45]

A variety of respiratory conditions, including shortness of breath, were also diagnosed and treated in other ancient Asian cultures. The classical system of Indian medicine, āyurveda (meaning literally 'knowledge for longevity'), was based on maintaining or restoring the balance between three bodily humours and seven bodily constituents. Recorded and transmitted in Sanskrit texts, āyurvedic treatments were predominantly herbal but, like Greek medicine, also included advice regarding exercise, diet, and sleep, as well as massage, enemas, and surgery. Although the dominance of this traditional Indian medicine was challenged to some extent by the assimilation of *ūnānī tibb*, a Galenic form of medical practice, into India from Islam in the eleventh century, both systems persisted within a pluralistic medical culture into the modern period.[46]

Within the ancient āyurvedic context that fashioned medicine in India and Sri Lanka in particular, various 'phlegm diseases' were well known: the accumulation of phlegm could cause colds, catarrh, sinusitis, hay fever, and asthma. According to the *Caraka Samhitā*, a central āyurvedic text supposedly transmitted from the Hindu god Brahma to the Vedic sage Atreya and subsequently compiled by the physician Caraka, asthma (or *tamaka swasa*) was aggravated by humid, cold weather and could cause considerable distress to patients.[47] As in the classical Greek tradition explicated by medieval authors, such diseases were complicated and often difficult to treat, since they could be exacerbated both by cold foods, such as milk, which stimulated the production of phlegm, and by hot foods and medicines. Remedies were aimed at calming the aroused humour, largely by adopting an appropriate lifestyle, and at expelling the phlegm through medicinal inhalations (or *dhūma*), which had been used to treat respiratory disorders in India from the fourth millennium BC. In particular, Indian practitioners advised smoking various forms of powdered *Datura*, containing stramonium, to alleviate asthmatic symptoms. Significantly, the inhalation of stramonium not only continued to be employed by doctors and their patients in India, but also eventually spread to the West, where medicated cigarettes were used by Marcel Proust and others well into the twentieth century.[48] As was the case with Greek, Roman, and Islamic approaches to asthma and other forms of troubled breathing, ancient Egyptian, Chinese, and Indian medical traditions thus persisted forcefully into the modern period.

Although it is impossible to determine precisely how many people suffered or died from asthma in the ancient and medieval worlds, regular discussions in medical texts suggest close professional and personal familiarity with the signs, symptoms, and natural history of the condition. In spite of differences in the details, most ancient and medieval cultures adopted strikingly similar approaches to the causes, classification, and treatment of disease. According to ancient Greek, Egyptian, Islamic, Jewish, Chinese, and Indian medicine, illness was routinely regarded as the product of imbalances in the quantity and flow of humours or their equivalent, generated by a combination of constitutional factors, inappropriate lifestyles, and environmental circumstances. The restoration of health demanded a return to physiological and spiritual equilibrium, achieved through close attention to lifestyle reinforced whenever necessary by the application of herbal remedies, the inhalation of smoke and vapours, blood-letting, purging, massage, acupuncture, and psychological and emotional support.

Within these broad philosophies of medicine, ancient and medieval clinicians recognized a range of breathing difficulties, which were increasingly described, at least in the West, in Greek terms: dyspnoea; tachypnoea; orthopnoea; and asthma. Although the boundaries between these conditions were indistinct, it is apparent that by the late-medieval period the term 'asthma' had been incorporated into many European languages and had developed a relatively fixed clinical persona. The word 'asthma' was first used in English in approximately 1398, and variants appeared in French, Spanish, German, Italian, and Portuguese.[49] In both Eastern and Western medical traditions, asthma was then understood to be caused by the accumulation of phlegm in the lungs leading to laboured wheezy breathing that was often worse at night, a cough, and the sensation of gasping for breath. While acute asthma attacks usually subsided within an hour or so, the potential for chronic asthma to lead to declining health and death was recognized and feared by doctors and sufferers alike.

The classical symptoms of asthma, faithfully captured by ancient and medieval writers, continued to trouble both patients and doctors through the Renaissance and early modern period. The fall of Constantinople in 1453 triggered a revival of Greek culture and the rediscovery of Greek and Roman texts throughout Western Europe. Transmitted through Hebrew and Arabic translations, many ancient medical and philosophical works became available in Latin printed editions for the first time and were sometimes bound together into a single textbook, known as the *Articella*, designed for the increasing numbers of students entering European, and particularly Italian, medical schools during the fifteenth, sixteenth, and seventeenth centuries: in addition to Latin translations of medieval treatises, the works of Galen were available in Latin from the late fourteenth century; editions of Seneca and Celsus appeared in the 1470s; and translations of Aretaeus were printed in the 1550s. However, while ancient Greek, Egyptian, Arabic, and Hebrew formulations of asthma certainly continued to influence modern understandings of the condition, new forms of scientific research and greater awareness of alternative medical traditions during the Renaissance and Enlightenment also facilitated the emergence of a cosmopolitan medicine that not only increasingly attempted to challenge ancient authorities by offering novel formulations of asthma, but also provided momentum for the eventual, if only partial, fusion of Eastern and Western medical wisdom.

II

ASTHMA REDEFINED

Robert Smith, aged 51, admitted a patient at the York County-Hospital, February 3, 1777, has been subject, for many years past, to an Asthma, particularly in the winter season, which has greatly weakened and impaired his constitution. Along with a cough, he is attacked in the night with a difficulty of breathing, which comes on suddenly, and continues with great violence for several hours. He complains too of want of sleep, constant thirst, head-ach, and soreness in his breast. His body is regular, pulse low, tongue clean, appetite bad, expectoration difficult.

Thomas Withers, *A Treatise on the Asthma*, 1786

I n 1552, the apparent superiority of new Italian modes of learning and investigation were adroitly demonstrated by the celebrated physician and mathematician Girolamo Cardano (1501–76). During the 1540s and early 1550s, John Hamilton (1511–71), the Roman Catholic archbishop of St Andrews who was a member of one of the most powerful families in Scotland and a prominent architect of church reform, had developed an increasingly severe and recalcitrant form of asthma, characterized by a cough, expectoration, and shortness

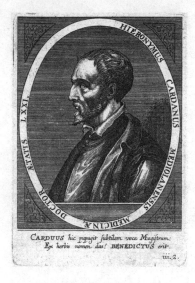

CARDUUS *hic pupugit subtilem voce Magistrum:*
Ex herbis nomen das! BENEDICTVS erit.
iii.2.

4. Girolamo Cardano, 1501–76.
(*Wellcome Library, London*)

of breath. Believing the condition to be the product of a cold, moist brain leading to the accumulation of phlegm, Hamilton's physician, Dr Cassanate, had tried in vain to restore his patient's health. Eventually, in September 1551, Cassanate wrote to Cardano imploring him to treat the archbishop. Having recently resigned from his position as Professor of Theoretical Medicine at Pavia, Cardano immediately accepted the invitation, met Cassanate in Lyons in February 1552, and arrived in Scotland in June that year.

Cardano was well placed to attend Hamilton. Although more famous for his mathematical works, such as *Ars magna*, in which he published solutions to cubic and quartic equations, Cardano was a renowned, if controversial, physician who had graduated in medicine from Padua in 1526. When he received Cassanate's request, Cardano was fortuitously studying Maimonides's treatise on asthma and developing his own theories about the condition. Cardano's close observation and examination of Hamilton over a period of six weeks reinforced his belief that the archbishop's asthma was due not to cold, moist humours, but to excessive heat precipitated by a life of luxury and venery, by the demands of work, and by his physician's misguided attempts to treat him in hot, smoky rooms. Accordingly, Cardano not only advised Hamilton to lead a more moderate, restrained, and restful lifestyle, but also prescribed a variety of remedies aimed at purging and cooling the body, including applying warm water to the head followed by cold-water showers, inhalations of elaterium, and applications of an ointment of tar, mustard, euphorbium (derived from a herb that is sometimes referred to as 'asthma weed'), honey of anthardus, and blister-fly to the skull. Cardano also insisted that Hamilton's mattress and pillows should not contain feathers, but be made of silk stuffed with dry straw and seaweed.

Cardano's regimen, carefully recorded in his *Consilia*, was immediately successful. The improvement in Hamilton's health was both dramatic and enduring and earned Cardano a substantial reward: when he left Scotland in September 1552 to return to Italy via London, Cardano received 1,800 crowns and a gold chain, in addition to the daily payment of twenty crowns during his stay. Significantly, Cardano's clinical acumen ultimately benefited him in other ways. After his son had been convicted and executed for murdering his unfaithful wife, Cardano's reputation declined: in 1563 he was dismissed from his Chair of Medicine at Pavia and exiled from Milan. Hounded for many years by the Inquisition, he was eventually arrested in Bologna in 1570 and imprisoned for heresy. In desperation, Cardano wrote to Archbishop Hamilton asking him to intervene on his behalf. Shortly before he was himself hanged by the enemies of Mary, Queen of Scots, Hamilton convinced the papal authorities that Cardano deserved clemency and successfully engineered the release of the physician who had largely cured his asthma twenty years previously.[1]

Although Cardano's treatment of Hamilton's asthma was clearly successful, it would be a mistake to regard his therapeutic interventions as evidence of a significant advance either in general theories of disease or in the specific treatment of asthma. As numerous sixteenth- and seventeenth-century medical treatises make clear, ancient understandings of asthma in terms of the accumulation of cold, moist humours persisted. Indeed, this was the main explanation for the prevalence of asthma, catarrh, and coughs amongst children, who were thought to have colder and moister temperaments than adults.[2] More particularly, it would be inappropriate to consider Cardano's rejection of feather mattresses as a precursor of later allergic theories of asthma, as some historians have suggested.[3] Cardano's preference for silk and straw merely reflected his belief in the need to avoid overheating the spine and brain. In this respect, Cardano's prescription was no more original than the formulations of asthma constructed by the ancient Greek physicians and the medieval Islamic and Jewish scholars on whom he self-consciously based his clinical approach. Like many other late-medieval and Renaissance humanist scholars in both France and Italy, Cardano was essentially subscribing to traditional Western theories of disease, according to which symptoms were the direct product of humoral imbalance. Within this conceptual framework, asthma constituted a particular form of breathing difficulty, triggered by excess phlegm and marked by wheezing, cough, and the sensation of choking.

Such continuity is also evident in parallel Eastern accounts of asthma. Seventeenth-century Chinese descriptions of the lung channel and its acupoints, which constituted locations on the body where acupuncture needles were inserted in order to treat a range of respiratory diseases including asthma and coughs, were largely based on ancient Daoist formulations of disease. Equally, the herbal medicine traditionally practised in *kanpō* clinics and derived from the ancient Chinese medical system remained at the heart of Japanese approaches to health and sickness even after the gradual infiltration and expansion of Western medicine from the end of the sixteenth century. In treating asthma, Japanese clinicians would often combine the two approaches: the gentle and systemic meridian treatments of orthodox *kanpō*, most notably herbal remedies but also massage, acupuncture, and moxibustion, would be employed to restore balance, while Western symptomatic treatments would be prescribed to manage localized respiratory features of the disease.

While continuity is evident in the evolution of ancient medical traditions, it is clear that during the Renaissance and early modern period European scholars in particular began to develop new approaches to the pathology and treatment of asthma, often referred to in this period as 'the asthma' or 'an asthma'. Innovations in theory and practice were initiated partly by developments in anatomy and partly by the increased international transmission of medical knowledge and practice generated by global travel. During the mid-sixteenth century, both tobacco and the native Brazilian plant ipecacuanha were imported into Europe from South America and became popular treatments for respiratory complaints. Similarly, travel to the East influenced the development of indigenous Chinese, Japanese, and Indian medicine and introduced a range of new therapeutic preparations to the Western medical pharmacopoeia. In addition to the gradual redefinition of asthma, there was another notable feature of early modern treatises on asthma. Although they were generally written in technical terms for a professional audience, many contemporary medical accounts were closely framed by personal experience: from the early seventeenth century through to the late nineteenth century, clinical descriptions of asthma were written almost exclusively by asthmatics.

Floyer's periodic asthma

Having grown disillusioned with his studies of law, mathematics, and astronomy, the Flemish nobleman Joan Baptista van Helmont (1579–1644) turned to medicine, successfully graduating from the University of Louvain in 1599. Although his support for various magical cures excited censure from both medical and theological scholars, van Helmont published extensively on a variety of clinical and scientific topics. Aligning himself initially with Paracelsus (1493–1541), van Helmont was critical of both Galenic medicine and Aristotelian philosophy. Instead, he constructed a complex system of the world, including health and disease, which was based on the action of *semina* (or seeds) directed by a spiritual entity, the *archeus*, and which linked mind, body, and soul: a disordered *archeus* allowed the *semina* of diseases to infiltrate and corrupt, and the aim of medicine was to restore the health and integrity of the *archeus*, thereby cleansing the body.

Van Helmont's major medical work, first published in Latin by his son in 1648 and translated into English in 1662, included a lengthy chapter on 'The Asthma or Stoppage of Breathing, and

Cough'. Himself an asthmatic, van Helmont immediately distanced himself from Hippocratic notions of phlegm descending from the brain to the lungs, emphasizing the failure of such ancient theories to furnish effective treatments. Although, like Hippocrates, he recognized similarities between asthma and epilepsy, referring to asthma at times as 'the falling-Sickness of the Lungs', van Helmont insisted that the disease generally originated in the lungs not the head: 'the *Lungs* is passable with pores or little holes, as long as we live…it is sufficiently manifest, that in the Asthma, there is a straightness of the same pores', ultimately caused in van Helmont's scheme by 'a Poysonous seed'. According to van Helmont, many traditional remedies such as the leaves or juice of coltsfoot and a linctus of fox lungs mixed with herbs, both of which were recommended for wheezing and shortness of breath by the English herbalist and astrologer Nicolas Culpeper (1616–54), served only to accentuate the symptoms by increasing the 'straightness' and obstruction of the air passages.[4]

From van Helmont's perspective, asthma occurred in two main forms, the first of which appeared only in women, the second in either sex: 'There is therefore, a two-fold asthma, one indeed Womanish, depending only on the government of the Womb, but the other is promiscuous, common to both sexes.'[5] While he rejected the possibility of humours flowing from the head, he suggested that the female form of asthma stemmed essentially from 'foul or stinking Vapours' ascending from the womb to block the pores in the lungs. Like the 'Head-aches and threatned Swoonings' to which women were supposedly susceptible, asthma in such patients was triggered by smells and fumes, strong emotions, and certain types of food and drink.

Van Helmont also described two separate clinical presentations of the disease, one a 'moist' asthma with the expectoration or 'spitting' of phlegm, the other a 'dry' asthma, although he recognized that in some patients a mixed form could occur. He illustrated these contrasting types with case histories that highlighted several distinctive features of the disease and that came to dominate early modern discussions of asthma. In the first place, he identified the manner in which both exposure to dust and eating 'Fishes fried with Oyl' could trigger asthma attacks. He also suggested that in some cases asthma originated in the stomach and could be suppressed or alleviated by a light diet: 'But a sparing Supper, as it gives rest to his Stomack; so also peace to his Lungs.' Another aspect noted by van Helmont was a familial association between asthma and skin complaints: he recounted the experiences of a man (and his mother and sister) who not only suffered from asthma, but who also 'itcheth throughout his whole body, casts off white Scales, and shews forth the likeness of a Leprousie'. Finally, he emphasized the idiosyncratic or capricious nature of asthma, noting that, while some women were distressed by sweet smells and sorrow, others remained unaffected.[6]

Van Helmont offered few remedies. He largely confined his comments on treatment to disparaging the cruelty or foolishness of previous approaches, offering in their place only the advice that, since the whole body was affected by the poisonous seed, the disease could be alleviated only by 'the Remedy of a Secret which may pierce all the paths of the Body throughout the whole, that it may leave nothing unattempted'.[7] In terms of both his rejection of humoral pathology and his resistance to ancient and medieval treatments, van Helmont was attempting to engineer a deliberate departure from classical approaches to asthma. While his formulations of disease were not routinely accepted, van Helmont clearly provided a constructive, if contentious, framework for subsequent disputes about the causes and manifestations of asthma.

Both the vibrancy and fragility of the revolutionary scientific agenda set by van Helmont and his contemporaries were made apparent by the work of two English physicians, Thomas Willis (1621–75) and John Floyer (1649–1734). Born in Wiltshire in 1621 but raised within the staunchly Royalist shadows of the University of Oxford, Willis saw his professional fortunes fluctuate with the fall and rise of the English monarchy. He initially struggled to establish a medical practice during the 1640s and 1650s, but his prospects improved partly as the result of the publication of a number of books on chemical medical philosophy and partly as the result of the restoration of Charles II in 1660, after which he was appointed Sedleian Professor of Natural Philosophy at Oxford. During the following years, Willis began his intricate studies of the anatomy of the brain and nerves, leading to the publication of *Cerebri anatome* in 1664 and *Pathologiae cerebri* in 1667, in which he provided detailed accounts of the distribution and action of nerves in both health and disease.

It was in his final work, *Pharmaceutice rationalis*, the first part of which was published in 1674, that Willis considered the causes, symptoms, and treatment of asthma. Although in this study, as in other publications, Willis attempted to set the practice of medicine on a new empirical and anatomical footing, shaped by developments in both morbid anatomy and chemistry, it is noticeable that, unlike van Helmont, he regularly appealed to ancient as well as modern authors, both in his general discussion of respiratory function and in his account of specific diseases such as asthma. Indeed, Willis's understanding of disease remained saturated by older notions of blood, humours, and spirits, as well as by more recent preoccupations with nerves and fibres.

Willis first established the anatomical and physiological features of the lungs and thorax. In particular, he noted that the 'Coats of the *Bronchia*, as also of the Larynx, have muscular Fibres of both kinds…from which we may also conclude, that all the lesser Pipes of the *Aspera Arteria* have their constant turns of Systole and Diastole, *viz*. all the Pipes are contracted while we breathe out, and relaxed while we suck in air'.[8] He also described the manner in which nerves were dispersed throughout the lungs, serving to regulate breathing, coughing, and laughing through their control of the diaphragm and thoracic muscles. Injury to any of these structures, or to the heart and pulmonary circulation, could result in breathing difficulties.

For Willis, asthma constituted a discrete and distinguishable condition marked by unrivalled respiratory distress:

> Among the Diseases whereby the Region of the breast is wont to be infested, if you regard their tyranny and cruelty, an Asthma (which sometimes by reason of a peculiar symptome is denominated likewise an Orthopnoea) does not deserve the last place; for there is scarce any thing more sharp and terrible than the fits hereof; the organs of breathing, and the precordia themselves, which are the foundations and Pillars of Life, are shaken by this disease, as by an Earthquake, and so totter, that nothing less than the ruine of the whole animal Fabrick seems to be threatned; for breathing, whereby we chiefly live, is very much hindred by the assault of this disease, and is in danger, or runs the risque of being quite taken away.[9]

In a passage which echoed van Helmont and heralded a growing division between humoral and nervous explanations of asthma, Willis described two principal forms of the condition.

In 'pneumonick' asthma, the 'passages bringing in the aire' were obstructed or not sufficiently open, as the result of 'thick humours and viscous, or purulent matter or blood extravasated' into the bronchi. Recognized and described by ancient authors, this brand of asthma could be triggered in patients predisposed to this condition by 'violent motion of the body or minde, excess of extern cold or heat, the drinking of Wine, Venery, yea sometimes mere heat of the Bed', as Cardano had previously intimated in his management of Archbishop Hamilton's asthma. By contrast, the 'convulsive' form of asthma, which, according to Willis, had not been acknowledged by classical authors, was caused by 'a defect or fault in the motive organs', and, more particularly, by 'morbific cause or matter' adversely affecting the muscular fibres, nerves, or brain. Some patients demonstrated a mixed clinical and pathological picture, especially if the asthma had become habitual.[10]

Although appropriate treatment might attenuate the fits and lengthen any periods of respite and although hot summer weather generally allowed asthmatics to breathe more freely, Willis, like many medical authors before him, regarded asthma as largely incurable. On occasions, it could also progress to more severe and potentially fatal conditions, such as dropsy and consumption. Nevertheless, Willis insisted that close attention to remedies aimed at either curing or preventing asthmatic fits was often beneficial. Curative strategies included a range of treatments that reflected his understanding of the causes and clinical presentations of asthma. In the first instance, Willis recommended simple measures to facilitate breathing, such as sitting upright in the fresh air, employing blood-letting and enemas to reduce plethora (an excess of blood or humours) and abdominal pressure, and administering 'pectoral Decoctions', such as the herbal resin gum ammoniacum, to promote expectoration and reduce catarrh. Secondly, he advised the use of anti-spasmodics, including preparations of the herbaceous plant asafoetida, to curtail asthmatic convulsions and anodynes to alleviate pain. In extreme cases, laudanum and other narcotics could be administered, albeit with caution, to sedate and suppress asthmatic spasms.[11] Between attacks, patients and physicians were advised to employ expectorants, anti-spasmodics, and purgatives, including the broth of 'an old cock', in order to restore the lungs, remove any 'morbific matter', and improve general health.

Willis concluded his reflections on asthma with a series of case histories, an approach that was gradually becoming the standard means of exemplifying clinical categories and substantiating medical theories. Over twenty years later, when John Floyer wrote probably the first treatise in English dedicated solely to asthma in 1698, he was able to adopt a slightly different and perhaps more convincing strategy, basing his recommendations and advice to patients and practitioners on over thirty years of battling against the disease himself. While Willis had certainly acknowledged the severity of the condition, pointing out that one of his patients felt himself to be 'in the agonie of death' during an asthmatic fit,[12] Floyer's personal experience of asthma and his first-hand knowledge of the efficacy (and, on occasions, inefficacy) of various treatments offered his readers more personal and more direct insights.

Born in Staffordshire in England in 1649, Floyer graduated in medicine from Oxford in 1680 before returning to Lichfield to practise as a physician until his death in 1734. Inspired largely by Galenic humoral principles, Floyer's published work incorporated a wide range of clinical and scientific interests: he published books on the classification of plant remedies, the preservation of health in old age, medical education, and cold-water bathing, which was sometimes recommended subsequently for asthmatics. In addition, impressed by traditional Chinese approaches to reading the pulse in order to establish a diagnosis, he devised a 'pulse watch' with a second hand for more accurate measurement of the heart rate. Throughout these works, Floyer expressed his scepticism of both the chemical theories proposed by van Helmont, Willis, and others, and the approaches adopted by empirics or quacks, who practised without a licence: 'pure Chymical Authors', he insisted in his treatise on asthma, 'know little of Anatomy, and the Nature of Animal Humours', and had unjustly rejected Galenic theories of humoral imbalances and cacochymias (or the unhealthy state of bodily fluids). Although Floyer acknowledged that Hippocrates and Galen had made occasional errors, he insisted that it was these 'old Writers' who had 'found out the most useful Medicines in the Asthma'.[13]

Floyer's *A Treatise of the Asthma* is a peculiar and complex work, which was translated into French and German and went through several highly popular and influential English editions. Written in an ornate, baroque style, the treatise is infused with evidence of Floyer's own pain and discomfort. The book is structured in four parts, setting out in turn the symptoms, the remote and accidental causes, and the treatments of asthma. Floyer's approach is evident from the introductory note to the reader. The purpose of respiration, he argued, was for 'preparing the Blood'. Breathing difficulties were caused by problems with the blood or in the heart, by obstruction of either the blood or air vessels by tumours, or by injury to the muscles of respiration

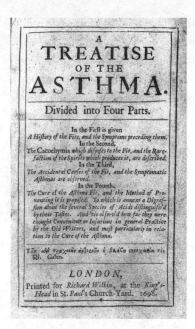

5. The title page of *A Treatise of the Asthma* (1698) by John Floyer. (*Wellcome Library, London*)

or to the 'spirits, moving those Muscles'. Within this scheme, asthma constituted a familiar figure of respiratory distress:

> WhentheMuscleslabourmuchforInspirationandExpiration, through some Obstruction, or Compression of the Bronchia, &c. we properly call this a Difficulty of Breath: But if this difficulty be by the Constriction of the Bronchia, 'tis properly the periodic Asthma: And if the Constriction be great, it is with Wheezing; but if less, the Wheezing is not so evident; the Pulse being stopt in the Asthma Fit, the Respiration is rare.[14]

Floyer divided asthma into two forms: 'continued Asthma' was largely the product of other disease processes, such as dropsy, empyema (the accumulation of pus in the pleural cavity), tubercles in the lungs, thoracic or abdominal tumours, and spinal conditions, which directly compressed the veins, the bronchi, or the nerves; 'periodic Asthma', by contrast, depended on bronchial constriction by 'windy Spirits', and occurred either after fevers, catarrh, and hypochondriacal fits or as the result of a 'flatulent Slimy Cacochymia, which is bred in the Stomach'. This latter form was the 'true Periodic flatulent Asthma', with which Floyer had been afflicted since childhood and which was the primary subject of his treatise.[15] Although Floyer acknowledged that very few patients died from periodic asthma attacks, some living in tolerable health for over fifty years, this form of the condition often induced consumptions, dropsies, lethargies, and inflammations that could prove fatal.

Floyer relied on his own personal diary of chronic asthma to convey the paradigmatic symptoms. The early signs of an attack were 'fulness of the stomach', an 'effervescence in the Blood' exacerbated by heat, a slight headache, and sleepiness. As night approached, the lungs of asthmatic patients began to feel 'rigid, stiff, or inflated', their heads seemed to be 'filled with Fumes, or Serous Humours', and they began 'to suck in their Breath, and wheeze a little': 'the Trachea, or its Bronchia', Floyer explained, 'have their Membranous and Nervous Fibres Contracted, by which the Wheezing is made in Expiration'. Although the patient might 'seem to have a Convulsive Cough before the Fit, and sometimes a little slimy Phlegm is spit up', Floyer was insistent that bronchial constriction was not primarily dependent on the accumulation of phlegm.[16]

Asthmatic fits proper usually began at around one or two o'clock in the morning, leading the patients to sit upright as breathing became more laboured and they struggled to breathe, cough, sneeze, spit, or speak freely. Respiratory efforts were impeded further by 'a great Inflation' of the membranes of the stomach, a 'rarefaction of its Contents', and a suffocating 'Flatuosity', sometimes followed by vomiting. At this stage, as the patient's pulse and temperature rose, the fit was exacerbated by the heat of a fire or by dust and smells. As the attack began to abate in the morning, the asthmatic might spit up some 'Gelly-like Phlegm'. Although in some cases a short 'Spitting Fit' of this nature might pass fairly rapidly, on many occasions attacks lasted several days, with phlegm being produced only from the third or fourth day, sometimes streaked with blood.[17]

Floyer carefully charted the periodicity of his own asthmatic attacks over seven years. He noticed that his asthma was both more frequent and more severe in the summer than the winter, that it frequently coincided with 'the Change of the Moon', probably as a result of accompanying alterations in the weather or wind direction, and that it varied according to location: while he was largely free from fits for twelve years in Oxford, he was immediately afflicted once he returned to his native Staffordshire. During the intervals between asthmatic fits, Floyer unsuccessfully tried a number of remedies to prevent relapse, including drinking pectorals such as gum ammonia-cum, tincture of lavender, and spirit of hartshorn to ease expec-toration, smoking amber with his tobacco, taking infusions of millipedes, being purged or bled, and drinking spa waters such as those at Bath. Finding none of these methods effective, Floyer found limited relief from vomiting once a month, and from tak-ing 'six Ounces of the *Cortex* infused in Wine' followed by 'three Ounces of *Ammoniacum*'. However, even these measures even-tually proved insufficient to prevent the return of asthmatic fits, prompting Floyer to reject the advice of most modern writers and to return to the 'rational Notions' of Galen and his medieval descendants.[18]

Although he reluctantly acknowledged a division between 'the Humid and the Old Hysteric *Asthma*' that authors such as Willis and van Helmont had promoted,[19] Floyer developed a typically idiosyncratic approach to the aetiology of the disease, locating the origins of the condition in 'an Effervescence in the Humours', which caused a 'Rarefaction of the Animal Spirits' leading in turn to a 'Preternatural State of the Chyle, and Blood, and Serum'. Dismissing purely chemical or mechanical approaches to the disease, Floyer argued that asthma was essentially a systemic condition in which the balance of all bodily fluids (blood, lymph, serum, and chyle, a milky fluid generated during digestion) was disturbed and the membranes of the stomach, lungs, and head were 'inflated' or rigidly expanded, leading to the range of abdominal symptoms, headaches, and drowsiness as well as breathlessness. Although he regarded asthma as a condition marked by slow, rather than fast, breathing, Floyer's overall account of the 'antecedent Cause' echoed many ancient descriptions of the disease:

> The Asthma is a high, slow, rare, and laborious Respiration, which depends immediately on the Inflation of the Membranes of the Lungs (which constrings the Bronchia, the Bladders of the Lungs and Blood Vessels) by windy Spirits, rarefied or propelled through the Glands of the Brain, either by external Accidents, or a periodic Febrile Effervescence of the Blood.[20]

From this broadly Hippocratic perspective, Floyer argued that the immediate triggers of asthma included any agent that encouraged 'a slow Effervescence, or Ebullition of our Blood', such as:

great Heats or Cold, violent Motions of the Body or Mind, any Excess in Eating and Drinking, or Venereal Pleasures; the Heat of the Bed, the Changes of the Weather to Rain, Snow, or from Frost to a Thaw; the Alteration of Clothes, the Changes of the Air at Spring and Fall: All these are causes of the Fever we call an Ephemera, and they also produce the Fits of the Asthma.[21]

In the third chapter of his treatise, Floyer explored these 'evident Causes' of asthma according to medieval notions of lifestyle or regimen. Moist air, 'fenny Vapours and Mists', the heat and smoke of fires, fumes, perfumes, and dust disturbed by sweeping a room or making a bed could all provoke asthmatic fits. While strong liquors and foods that generated a 'viscid Chyle' were to be avoided, 'a frugal and simple Diet' often prevented attacks. Exercise was known to trigger an asthmatic fit, but gentle exercise between fits was beneficial. Anger, fear, shouting, and excessive study produced asthma by inflaming 'the Spirits' and quickening the pulse, while regular purges, bleedings, and vomiting could help to restore the evacuations to normal and sometimes relieve or palliate, if not cure, a fit. Since fits often began during sleep, 'when the Nerves are filled with windy Spirits', narcotics were to be used only in moderation, preferably in conjunction with an acid, to 'compress the Inflations'.

Floyer also considered those conditions that produced asthma as a symptom, in some cases proving fatal: suppression of the menses; plethora; a polypus in the heart or lungs; coagulation of chyle or stones in the lungs; peripneumonia, a form of inflammation in and around the lungs; cachexia and other wasting diseases; 'a long Catarrh', often regularly occurring at 'great Changes of the Year', giving rise to what Floyer termed an 'Anniversary Asthma' in patients predisposed to the condition;

fevers; smallpox; spinal deformities; abdominal tumours, provoking a 'spurious Asthma'; and 'Cephalic Diseases', such as
apoplexy, gout, delirium, and hysterical fits.

Floyer's discussion of the causes of asthma concluded with
reflections on the differences between 'the Spitting and Hysterical Asthma'. While he acknowledged, like others before him,
that asthma expressed itself in distinct ways in different patients,
he was insistent that the two presentations were essentially
manifestations of a single pathology, marked in both cases by
constriction of the bronchi. While the origins of the two types
differed, one arising in the lungs and the other in the nerves, the
immediate triggers of the asthmatic fits in each case were identical, and in practice the two forms often merged, as patients with
dry, hysterical asthma often began to spit phlegm.[22]

Floyer's approach to treatment was also essentially medieval.
In particular, his advice focused on establishing a suitable regimen guided by close attention to the non-naturals. During the
asthmatic fit, patients were to avoid fumes and smells and sit
upright in an airy room to facilitate breathing. Vomiting, bleeding, blisters, and cool liquors were to be administered to abate
and compress the 'windy Spirits' and relieve bronchial constriction, and gentle opiates could be prescribed for bedtime.
Drawing heavily on Galen, Floyer recommended that, like the
diet, any medicines should be 'contrary to the Disease', that is
'of a cooling, attenuating, carminative Temper, not spirituous,
windy, viscid'. In particular, vinegar acids, renowned for their
therapeutic properties since the time of Hippocrates, were
thought to be effective in alleviating the inflammation and suffocation of asthmatic paroxysms.

Prevention demanded a combination of remedies for
maximum effect. Citing many ancient and medieval authors,

including Celsus, Galen, Oribasius, and Ibn Sīnā, Floyer recommended a range of decoctions, emetics, purgatives, digestives, sudorifics, and enemas to maintain respiratory health and reduce the frequency and severity of attacks. One of his favourite remedies, both for preventing and for alleviating asthma, was vinegar of squills, which was prepared from the bulbs of the sea onion and which had, according to Galen, been discovered originally by Pythagoras. As ancient authors such as Hippocrates were aware, the acrid taste of vinegar preparations could be moderated by the addition of honey, thereby generating 'oxymel of squills', a treatment that had also been advocated by Willis. Although Floyer recognized the side effects of vinegar of squills, its broad range of actions made it a favoured tool in the early modern battle against asthma.[23]

It is tempting to regard the publication of Floyer's monograph as a pivotal moment in the history of asthma: comprising an extensive overview of the causes, diagnosis, pathology, and treatment of the condition, *A Treatise of the Asthma* was often cited and quoted by subsequent authors, becoming a standard, if sometimes contested, reference point for all modern Western discussions of the disease. However, Floyer's reliance on ancient and medieval texts and on traditional remedies, combined with his aggressive dismissal of modern therapeutic fashions, suggests that the light of ancient Greek, Islamic, and Jewish medicine had not yet been extinguished. While the revolutionary process set in motion by van Helmont and Willis certainly began to gather momentum during the eighteenth century as an expanding medical marketplace provided opportunities for the proliferation of novel theories and treatments, Floyer's intimate study of asthma testifies to the continued relevance of Galen and his followers for the course of modern medicine.

Enlightenment models

In 1717, the French composer Marin Marais (1656–1728) published his fourth book of pieces for the bass viol or viola da gamba. The second part of the book comprised a single long composition of thirty-six pieces 'of great difficulty', entitled *Suitte d'un goût étranger*. Like most baroque suites, Marais's work included a variety of allemandes, sarabandes, courantes, gigues, and other dance forms, some of which were given descriptive titles. Buried in the midst of the *Suitte*, but without any indication as to why the piece was given this particular title, was the 'Allemande l'asmatique', written in quadruple time in G major and, like most allemandes, incorporating two refrains, each played twice. Although some of Marais's allemandes were serious and stately, placing great technical demands on the performer, the 'Allemande l'asmatique' constituted one of his lighter dances, in which the tempo was faster and the melody less burdened by chords and contrapuntal devices. Intended perhaps to reflect the wheezes, or what became known as the musical *râles*, of asthmatics, the 'Allemande l'asmatique' was to be played 'Tres gay'.[24]

The light-hearted elegance of Marais's lyrical asthma stood in stark contrast to contemporary personal and medical accounts of the disease, which increasingly stressed its gravity and potential fatality. In his extensive survey of the diseases of workers published in Latin in 1713, the Italian physician Bernadino Ramazzini (1633–1714) had described the impact of exposure to dust on bakers and millers, who became 'finally asthmatic' (*asthmatici*), and on the sifters and measurers of grain, who became 'short of breath [*anhelosi*] and cachectic and rarely reach old age', as their lungs became irritated and they eventually choked from the

Allemande L'Asmatique

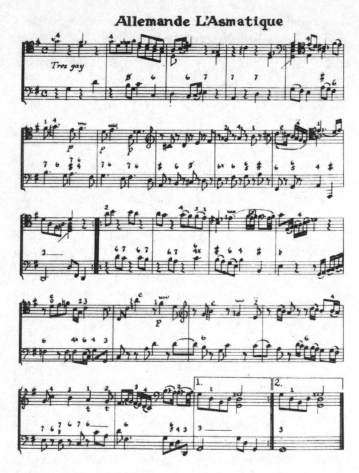

6. 'Allemande l'asmatique', composed in 1717 by Marin Marais.

continued inhalation of fine particles of flour and wheat.[25] Over subsequent decades, both medical writers and asthma sufferers regularly emphasized the manner in which asthma could debilitate and kill. Although precise figures of deaths from asthma are not available from this period, medical authors insisted that death from asthma was possible, particularly if other respiratory conditions supervened or if childhood asthma was left untreated. In 1778, the English Methodist preacher Thomas Maxfield (d. 1784) substantiated these beliefs by publishing an account of the spiritual life of his wife, Elizabeth, who had 'died of an Asthma' the previous year. Triggered by a 'violent cold' some fourteen or fifteen years before her death, Elizabeth's asthma had gradually worsened until 'she could hardly breathe' and struggled to speak. During her final hours, 'she continued in great pain thro' shortness of breath' and became increasingly weak 'as she never lay down from Thursday morning till she was laid down a corps'.[26]

The fear of incapacity and death haunted other contemporary accounts of asthma. In 1766, the Scottish surgeon Tobias Smollett (1721–71), popular author of *The Adventures of Roderick Random* and *The Adventures of Peregrine Pickle*, published a detailed account of his travels with his wife through France and Italy following the tragic death of their daughter. On several occasions he was concerned that prolonged exposure to cold and rain combined with the exhaustion of their journey would provoke 'a terrible fit of the asthma'. Smollett's anxieties proved unfounded, as the 'hard exercise of mind and body' during his travels apparently served to improve his health by counteracting the 'relaxation of the fibres' and curbing the 'listlessness, indolence, and dejection of the spirits' supposedly induced by his previously sedentary lifestyle.[27]

As Smollett's account suggests, while contemporary authors lamented the privations of asthma, Enlightenment ideologies of disease brought fresh hopes of relief. During the late seventeenth and early eighteenth centuries, as novel methods of investigation and innovative formulations of disease spread across Europe following the scientific revolution, patients and doctors alike displayed a renewed faith in the ability of science and technology to improve society and to classify and cure disease. Eager to reject older irrational, mystical models of health and sickness, prominent Enlightenment physicians, such as Thomas Sydenham (1624–89), Georg Stahl (1660–1734), Friedrich Hoffmann (1660–1742), and Herman Boerhaave (1668–1738), not only increasingly emphasized the importance of careful observation of the patterns and presentations of disease, but also strove to develop 'a simple and logical synthesis of medical knowledge designed to replace increasingly obsolete humoral conceptions inherited from antiquity' and to alleviate or conquer ill health.[28] Combined with a competitive patronage system and a greater degree of social mobility and consumer choice, Enlightenment thought encouraged the proliferation of speculative, and often mutually exclusive, medical systems, which emphasized the mechanical behaviour of bodily fluids, the centrality of digestive chemistry, the role of the soul or 'anima', or increasingly the functions of the nervous and muscular systems in maintaining health and causing disease.

The immediate impact of these theoretical shifts was a transitory fragmentation of previous theories of asthma and the proliferation of new treatments. During the early decades of the eighteenth century, a variety of individual approaches emerged, many of which, ironically, reproduced ancient humoral accounts of disease or reinforced a reliance on regimen. In 1729, for example, the author of *An Enquiry into the Causes of the Present Epidemical Diseases* insisted that conditions such as fevers, coughs, catarrhs, asthma, and rheumatisms were collectively the product of the 'Insalubrity of the Air', leading to the retention and accumulation of phlegm in those patients predisposed to these conditions by their inheritance. If the retained 'Matter seizes on the Lungs', it created 'an asthmatick Cough or Shortness of Breath', which, if untreated, could develop into a 'settled *Asthma*'. In some cases, medical authors also drew heavily on Eastern, and particularly Chinese, approaches to medicine to expand the Western pharmacopoeia. As the popularity of both Floyer's work on the pulse and Jean-Baptiste du Halde's *General History of China* suggest, Chinese medicine and culture were increasingly in vogue across Europe during the eighteenth century. One outcome of this *chinoiserie* was the recommendation of Chinese recipes for asthma that incorporated Gin seng, Fou tse, Sou meon, and various teas.[29]

During the 1750s, the English physician and actor John Hill (d. 1775) denounced contemporary obsessions with such exotic remedies. Criticizing physicians for unnecessarily ransacking Africa 'for its nauseous Ammoniacum to give breath in Asthmas', Hill suggested that effective remedies were often to be found much closer to home. Italian or English spring honey, for example, taken regularly and sometimes in conjunction with the perennial herb erysimum, not only cured asthmatic fits but also prevented their return. Interestingly, according to Hill, while honey provided a 'certain cure' for the 'real Asthma', it was ineffective in the 'convulsive Asthma', which was 'altogether a different distemper, it is really a nervous complaint; and has only been called an Asthma, because the symptoms, particularly the difficulty of breathing, in some degree resemble an Asthma'.[30]

Hill's dismissal of convulsive asthma as a spurious form of the disease ran counter to a growing conviction that the condition was primarily a nervous one. Although some writers continued to identify a wide range of different types and causes of asthma, most late Enlightenment medical authorities regarded asthma in more simple terms as a single species generated by a disordered or irritated nervous system. In his internationally acclaimed *Domestic Medicine*, first published in 1769, the Scottish physician William Buchan (1728–1805) echoed many of his peers when he attempted to guard readers 'against the destructive influences of Ignorance, Superstition, and Quackery'. Committed to diffusing 'medical knowledge among the people', Buchan characterized asthma as a disease of the lungs that, contrary to the claims of empirics and quacks, was seldom cured. Like many authors before him, Buchan distinguished between humoral and nervous forms. Caused by hereditary factors as well as fumes, violent exercise, the 'obstruction of customary evacuations', or 'violent passions of the mind', asthma was treated with a suitable regimen, which might include travel to a warmer climate for those who could afford it, as well as a variety of familiar medicines: expectorants such as oxymel of squills and gum ammoniac for 'the moist asthma'; or anti-spasmodics such as paregoric elixir, comprising a camphorated tincture of opium, and Peruvian or Jesuit's bark, introduced into Europe from Peru in the seventeenth century, for 'the convulsive or nervous asthma'. Buchan also advocated a 'very strong infusion of roasted coffee' as a means of relieving an asthmatic paroxysm.[31]

Buchan's simple scheme was reinforced and refined by his compatriot, William Cullen (1710–90). Born in Hamilton in 1710, Cullen was initially apprenticed to a surgeon apothecary in Glasgow, but moved to London in 1729 and worked for a period as a ship's surgeon. Returning to Scotland in 1732, Cullen established a private practice in his home town and lectured in chemistry at the University of Glasgow, before moving to Edinburgh

University, where he was appointed first to the chair in chemistry and subsequently to the chair in the theory of medicine. In line with many of his contemporaries, Cullen was particularly interested in the classification of disease, or nosology. Within this context, Cullen's *Practice of Physic*, which was published in four volumes between 1777 and 1784 and was translated into most European languages, has been described as 'both a culmination and the swansong of Enlightenment medicine', serving to consolidate the 'systematic, nosological approach based primarily on symptoms' that was characteristic of the period.[32]

Although Cullen divided diseases into four main categories—namely, fevers, wasting diseases, neuroses, and local diseases—he was particularly interested in the manner in which disorders of the nervous system played a central role in disease causation. His neuropathological approach shaped not only his diagnosis but also his approach to treatment. In addition, his preoccupation with the nervous system was linked to wider Enlightenment anxieties about the impact of modern civilization on health. Echoing the earlier fears of George Cheyne (1671–1743), who had regarded asthma as one of a range of modern 'nervous distempers', including spleen, vapours, lowness of spirits, colic, gout, and rheumatism, which were induced by overindulgence and inactivity,[33] Cullen explained the apparent rise of chronic nervous diseases in terms of the greater sensibility of Western civilized nations, wrought partly by constitutional factors such as race, class, gender, and age, and partly by luxurious, sedentary, and intemperate lifestyles.

Within Cullen's classification of disease, asthma constituted a form of dyspnoea or breathing difficulty caused primarily by 'an affection of the nervous system', rather than by the accumulation of mucus, which was characteristic of 'Dyspnoea

Catarrhalis' rather than asthma. Distancing himself from common usage of the word to denote 'every case of difficult breathing', Cullen insisted that the term 'asthma' should properly be confined to cases previously referred to as 'Spasmodic Asthma' or 'Asthma Convulsivum'. True asthma, Cullen insisted, was often hereditary, affected men more than women, and usually appeared first at, or after, puberty. Cullen's succinct description of asthma attacks echoed those of many physicians and sufferers before him:

> At whatever time they come on, it is for the most part suddenly, with a sense of tightness and stricture across the breast, and a sense of straitness in the lungs impeding inspiration. The person thus attacked, if in a horizontal situation, is immediately obliged to get into somewhat of an erect posture, and requires a free and cool air. The difficulty of breathing goes on for some time increasing, and both inspiration and expiration are performed slowly, and with a wheezing noise. In violent fits, speaking is difficult and uneasy. There is often some propensity to coughing, but it can hardly be executed.[34]

According to Cullen, fits of asthma, which often continued for several nights and tended to recur throughout life, could be triggered particularly by external heat, sudden changes in the weather, exercise, a full meal, 'passions of the mind', odours, smoke, and dust. The proximate cause of the fits, he argued, was 'a preternatural, and in some measure a spasmodic, constriction of the muscular fibres of the bronchiae; which not only prevents the dilatation of the bronchiae necessary to a free and full inspiration, but gives also rigidity which prevents a full and free expiration'.[35] However, while Cullen's supposedly modern approach highlighted the role of the nervous and muscular systems, his explanation of the remote causes of asthma and related nervous conditions, such as

hysteria, hypochondria, dyspepsia, and gout, carried distant rever-
berations of Floyer: 'This preternatural constriction, like many
other convulsive and spasmodic affections, is readily excited by a
turgescence of the blood, or other cause of any unusual fulness
and distension of the vessels of the lungs.'[36]

Although asthma could sometimes prove fatal if it was complicated by phthisis (a form of tuberculous consumption) or by
an aneurysm of the heart or great vessels, and although asthma
attacks often threatened 'immediate death', most patients with
asthma 'lived long under this disease' according to Cullen.
However, asthma was rarely entirely cured. Since the disease
was inherited and idiosyncratic, the best hope lay in identifying and avoiding any occasional or exciting causes, including
tea and coffee, which weakened the 'nerves of the stomach'.
While the blood-letting, purging, vomiting, and acids recommended by Floyer and others might alleviate the disease and
while a light diet and gentle exercise might prevent relapse,
Cullen argued that the patient's greatest source of relief was the
consumption of anti-spasmodics, the most powerful of which
was opium. Any concerns about the safety of narcotics were,
in Cullen's eyes, the result of failing to distinguish adequately
'between certain plethoric and inflammatory cases of dyspnoea, improperly named Asthma, and the genuine spasmodic
asthma we treat of here'.[37]

Cullen's classification of asthma as a form of neurosis and
his prescription for its effective treatment were substantially
extended in a full-length treatise on the subject published in
1786 by Thomas Withers (1750–1809), physician to the York
County Hospital. Like Cullen, Withers focused largely on convulsive asthma. Drawing on his extensive experience as a hospital physician at the Edinburgh Royal Infirmary, at St Thomas's

Hospital in London, and at York, as well as on his private practice and treatment of poorer dispensary patients, Withers was
dismissive of most previous scholarship: Floyer's treatise was
useful, but 'full of false theory, vague hypotheses, contradic-
tory opinions, and ridiculous practice'; the work of John Millar,
who had suggested in 1769 that asthma 'fell principally upon the
lower class of people',[38] was 'short and imperfect'; Boerhaave
had 'no distinct notion of the disease'; and ancient authors such
as Hippocrates and Galen were 'confused and unintelligible'.
Only William Cullen's lectures on the role of the nervous system offered Withers any constructive insights.[39]

Withers's treatise provides a rare impression of the prevalence
of asthma during the eighteenth century. The frequency of the
condition, he argued, had recently 'greatly engaged the attention of the medical faculty'. Although asthma had been known,
albeit imperfectly, to ancient writers, Withers was in no doubt
that this disease was 'more frequent in the present æra, than it
formerly were'. Like many parallel contemporary accounts of
chronic conditions, Withers attributed the rise in asthma to the
perils of modern living: 'The greater irritability and weakness of
the constitution in these days, may, in some measure, account
for the greater frequency of the Asthma, especially if we add the
inventive genius, and the rapid progress of mankind in all the
various arts of modern luxury and refinement.'[40] Along with
gout and other nervous conditions, asthma had been effectively
reformulated by Enlightenment physicians as one of the cardinal diseases of civilization.

Like Cullen, Withers was keen to clarify the meaning of the
term. Although he acknowledged that some patients presented
with 'the *humoural* or *spitting Asthma*', also sometimes referred to
as 'senile' asthma because it was more common in the elderly,

he preferred to apply the term more strictly to Cullen's nervous, convulsive, or spasmodic form of the condition. However, Withers drew the line between the two forms of the disease less securely than Cullen. Prolonged asthma, Withers argued, induced chronic weakness, which in turn not only exacerbated the impact of the disease but also altered the clinical manifestations. As the disease progressed, the patient's anxiety deepened and, like Seneca many centuries before, 'he labours in respiration, as if every moment would be his last'. Moreover, with time, the overproduction of phlegm increased, producing shortness of breath even in the absence of an asthmatic attack and blurring the boundary between nervous and humoral asthma: 'Thus the *humoral Asthma* is united with the convulsive, and both together exist in the same patient.'[41]

Withers's discussion of the immediate causes of asthma attacks was also more elaborate and more fluid than Cullen's, acknowledging the role of both an increased sensitivity of the muscular fibres of the bronchi and the overproduction of mucus. The abruptness and relatively short duration of attacks and the tendency to recover rapidly before any significant expectoration of phlegm suggested that 'sudden contraction of the muscular coats of the air vessels of the lungs' was the primary convulsive factor, a supposition apparently supported by anatomists. However, when humoral asthma supervened, alterations in the mucous glands contributed to the clinical picture: 'Hence the proximate cause of the convulsive Asthma, when complicated with the humoral, (which, as we have observed, is the most common state in which it appears) is a *spasmodic contraction* of the air-vessels of the lungs, preceded and followed by a *relaxation* of the mucous glands, with an *encreased secretion* of mucus.'[42]

More remote causes of the disease included a familiar range of occasional triggers, such as cold foggy weather, dust, the smell of a new feather bed, fatigue, violent exercise, strong emotions, and intemperance, which largely operated by weakening the nervous system, as well as a variety of predisposing causes, including a narrow contracted chest, a '*morbid irritability of the lungs*', or some form of pulmonary obstruction as the result of other disease processes. Significantly, irritability of the lungs was rarely natural but far more often acquired. Echoing earlier formulations of asthma by Cardano, Ramazzini, and others, Withers suggested that 'the chief cause of this acquired irritability is *artificial external heat*, accumulated about the body by means of *fires, cloathing*, and *houses*'. Prolonged overexposure to heat rendered bodies more susceptible to sudden changes in the temperature, explaining the prevalence of asthma amongst cooks, bakers, blacksmiths, and brewers: 'This class of men, pale, sallow, and often emaciated, is more subject to the Asthma than any other.' However, while such lower-class occupations predisposed many to the disease, those most at risk were patients in the 'middling as in the higher stations of life', who possessed the 'greatest delicacy of constitution'.[43]

According to Withers, asthma was an obstinate complaint, which was difficult, but not impossible, to cure and which could be fatal. His approach to treatment of the fits followed traditional lines: the practitioner's aim was to alleviate spasm, promote expectoration, and mitigate any urgent symptoms. To this end, Withers devised a suitable regimen according to the patient's age, constitution, and habits, which he then reinforced with bleeding, expectorants, emetics, laxatives and purgatives, anti-spasmodics such as musk, camphor, castor, asafoetida, and opium, and tonics such as Peruvian Bark, bitters, and the

Flowers or Calx of Zinc, which contained zinc oxide. This latter class of remedies was of particular interest to Withers, who suggested that their efficacy in cases of convulsive asthma had not been sufficiently recognized. Having started using Flowers of Zinc in 1776 on the grounds that it often proved beneficial in other spasmodic disorders, Withers was rapidly impressed by its utility, employing it on numerous occasions to reduce spasm and strengthen the patient's constitution. Many of the preparations recommended by Withers were patent medicines, such as James's Powder, which contained phosphate of lime and oxide of antimony and had been formulated by the Staffordshire-born physician Robert James (1705–76). Significantly, antimony in the form of emetic tartar, which was liberally prescribed for George III during his episodes of madness, was also regularly recommended for asthma.[44]

Prevention during remission relied largely on employing the same remedies. In addition to the regular use of the specific medicinal preparations capable of treating an acute attack, patients were advised to adopt a healthier lifestyle. This might include moving to the country or perhaps to a warmer climate for purer air, eating a plain and moderate diet, bathing in cold or temperate waters, wearing cool clothing, ensuring adequate domestic ventilation, and avoiding occasional causes of asthma such as 'the smell of new feather-beds'. Ultimately, cure required patients to 'cast off the effeminacy of the present times, abandon the destructive luxury of heat, and compelled by unanswerable reasons and long experience, return to follow that line of conduct, which Providence originally intended for us, and which alone is suited to the nature and structure of our constitutions'.[45]

The final two-thirds of Withers's treatise comprised fifty detailed case histories enriched by his own observations and reflections. As the case books and diaries of contemporary provincial doctors suggest, collections of cases offered an ideal medium for teaching and refining clinical skills; the Leeds surgeon William Hey (1736–1819), for example, kept detailed records of cases treated, including notes on several asthma patients, both for his own personal use and for instructing students and apprentices.[46] Prefaced by quotes from Hippocrates and Seneca, Withers's clinical accounts served particularly to demonstrate the value of his preferred remedies for effecting a cure in otherwise intractable circumstances. Although the cases were apparently selected from a much larger number, they give some provisional sense of the character and distribution of asthma in the late eighteenth century. Of the fifty patients, most of whom were treated for a period of several weeks as either in-patients or out-patients at the York County Hospital between 1776 and 1785, twenty-six were male and twenty-four were female. Although the majority of Withers's patients were adults, their ages on admission to hospital or on first consultation ranged from 7 weeks to 62 years old; as Withers pointed out, asthma was not uncommon in young children and in these cases was often precipitated by an infection such as whooping cough or measles.

Most of Withers's patients appear to have suffered from a mixed form of the condition, in which convulsive asthma was complicated by a humoral or catarrhal component. By the end of the eighteenth century, it would appear that this image of asthma as a condition caused primarily by periodic bronchial constriction, with or without the overproduction of mucus, was largely accepted. As a result, treatment focused increasingly on the role of anti-spasmodics, bolstered by a suitable regimen. However, as Withers himself acknowledged, this theory of asthma lacked supporting evidence from post-mortem examinations. Indeed, he explicitly warned his readers that future investigations might reveal alternative explanations:

> It is worth attention, for probably it may be hereafter found, that some species of the Asthma may originate from a disease in those mucous glands of the bronchia which secrete that bluish or grey-colored mucus, and be afterwards communicated more or less to the substance of the lungs themselves. Nothing but frequent dissections of dead bodies can clear up this point, nor indeed many others in the science of medicine, which are still involved in darkness and uncertainty.[47]

As Withers knew, the post-mortem findings in patients who had died from asthma were often unrevealing. In his account of a 50-year-old woman treated at a dispensary, Withers included a brief discussion of the case of John Strickney, whose asthma had deteriorated following his admission to hospital in July 1780, leading to his death approximately one month later. Although the post-mortem identified some water in the abdomen and chest, suggestive of 'an universal dropsy', the lungs and other viscera 'appeared to be not much diseased'.[48] Similar observations about the limits of post-mortem evidence had been made by John Millar in 1769, who pointed out not only that findings at dissection varied according to the stage of the disease and the degree of mucus production, but also that such evidence needed to be interpreted carefully in the context of the clinical history.[49] Indeed, as increasing numbers of dissections were carried out in European hospitals from the late eighteenth century onwards under the auspices of a new, topographical morbid anatomy, they initially tended to challenge Cullen's methodical nosological formulation of asthma as primarily a spasmodic, nervous condition.

Dissecting asthma

The forms and boundaries of pathological anatomy were largely forged by continental European physiologists and pathologists during the late eighteenth and nineteenth centuries. Early interest in locating the anatomical sites of various diseases was evident in the work of Giovanni Battista Morgagni (1682–1771) and his Italian peers, who attempted to correlate clinical symptoms with autopsy findings. Stimulated partly by Morgagni's *De sedibus et causis morborum*, published in 1761, the quest to determine the origins of diseases at the level of organs and tissues spread rapidly. In Britain, Matthew Baillie (1761–1823) employed extensive post-mortem evidence to provide clear descriptions of the pathology of numerous clinical conditions, including cirrhosis, emphysema, and pneumonia. His major work, *Morbid Anatomy of Some of the Most Important Parts of the Human Body*, first published in 1793, was translated into many European languages and appeared in several English and American editions. The finest and most influential exponent of the new localized pathology, however, was the French surgeon Marie-François-Xavier Bichat (1771–1802). Although he accepted that some conditions, notably nervous diseases and fevers, were not addressed adequately in his system of investigation, Bichat's *Traité des membranes* (1799) and *Anatomie générale* (1801) provided an innovative conceptual and practical framework for exploring the anatomical and histological basis of disease.

It is significant that, while his classification of diseases was based primarily on systematic analysis of the symptoms experienced by patients and the signs observed or elicited by physicians, William Cullen was not opposed to the art of pathology, acknowledging that the 'dissection of morbid bodies is one of the best means of improving us in the distinction of diseases'.[50] However, it is evident that the new pathological anatomy that emerged around the dawn of the nineteenth century began to undermine many of Cullen's nosological assumptions. In particular, Cullen's formulation of asthma as primarily a spasmodic nervous condition characterized by periodic bronchial constriction became a subject of increasingly intense debate amongst European and North American physicians.

In 1797, Robert Bree (1758–1839), an English physician born in Warwickshire, published A Practical Inquiry into Disordered Respiration. Like Floyer, Bree was plagued with chronic asthma, leading to his early retirement from practice in Leicester in 1793. Having spent some time in the army in East Anglia, where his asthma improved, Bree returned to practice in 1796, when he was appointed physician to the Birmingham General Hospital. Ten years later he moved to London, where he became a Fellow of the Royal College of Physicians and a Fellow of the Royal Society, served as vice-president of the Medical and Chirurgical Society, and treated the Duke of Sussex for asthma. In addition to the Practical Inquiry, which appeared in an extended edition in 1800, Bree also published on consumption and cholera.

Bree's inquiry was largely provoked by his opposition to Cullen's speculative 'Spasmodic theory'. At a broad level, he warned his readers that the proliferation of medical theories built on precarious hypotheses that were unsupported by historical authorities or pathological investigations constituted 'one cause of the turn for quackery that infests this country'. Most writers on asthma since Willis, he argued, had involved themselves in such conjecture: 'Asthma has been more subjected to the caprice of hypothesis and prevailing theories, than any others whose appearances could be as distinctly traced to a material exciting cause.'[51] At a more specific level, Bree was convinced that neither evidence from dissections nor clinical experience supported Cullen's assertion that asthma was caused by nervous contraction of the bronchi. While convulsive contractions of the muscles of respiration were certainly evident in asthmatics, there was as yet no proof of bronchial constriction. Moreover, although the doctrines of Floyer and Cullen had been routinely accepted, they had so far failed to furnish physicians or patients with effective cures.

Bree suggested an intriguing alternative understanding and classification of asthma, founded in part on much earlier formulations of the condition. Just as spasmodic contractions of the gut were caused by irritation and were aimed at removing any noxious material 'for the safety of the body', so convulsive contractions of the respiratory muscles in asthma essentially operated 'to relieve the internal functions from injury or interruption'. Asthma thus constituted a protective mechanism to preserve the integrity and health of the lungs. Any material irritation or the presence of another medical condition affecting the lungs, such as hydrothorax, empyema, tumours, and gibbosity (a marked curvature of the spine), could produce what Floyer had termed 'continued' asthma. However, on the basis that the diaphragm and abdominal muscles operated in sympathy 'as common instruments of relief', it was also possible that irritation of either the lungs, with fumes, dust, and the accumulation of mucus, or the abdominal viscera was capable of inducing a symptomatic form of continued asthma.[52]

In cases similar to Floyer's periodic flatulent asthma or Cullen's spasmodic asthma, where the source of irritation was not readily apparent, Bree suggested that asthmatic convulsions were often preceded by dyspepsia, flatulence, and distention of the stomach and bowels. As the attack developed, the characteristic symptoms appeared: difficulty breathing; a sense of 'straitness in the chest'; wheezing; and a cough, leading to copious expectoration of mucus towards the end of the fit. In essence, the cause of such paroxysms was the same as in continued asthma: the respiratory and abdominal muscles were labouring to remove or overcome a local irritant, particularly mucus. Drawing on ancient Greek, Roman, and Arabian authorities, as well as his own experience, Bree argued that the accumulation of, and physiological attempt to remove, mucus from the lungs should be regarded as a principal cause of the disease. One of Cullen's errors was his failure to recognize the weight of historical evidence.

Bree attempted to support his theory with evidence from dissections. Although uncomplicated asthma was rarely fatal, it was possible to examine the lungs of asthmatics who had died from unrelated acute disorders. Citing the post-mortem findings of Morgagni, Baillie, Millar, and others, as well as the results of experiments on animals, Bree argued that the lungs of asthmatics were regularly marked by effusions of serum and mucus from 'capillary vessels, greatly weakened by remote causes' into the trachea, bronchi, and smaller air spaces, but by no evidence of bronchial constriction. In such cases, the 'line of separation' between spasmodic asthma and catarrh, and indeed between so-called humoral and convulsive forms of asthma, was thus lost:

> If the tone of the exhalents of the lungs be greatly reduced in a habit predisposed to a ready association of muscles, and particularly of morbid contractions of the respiratory muscles, Asthma may be the disease occasioned by the defluxion, which, in other subjects, might be called Suffocative Catarrh.[53]

Having catalogued a series of more specific objections to Cullen's theory of spasmodic bronchial constriction, Bree concluded the second edition of his work with a concise summary of his position and a series of case histories. Arguing that all forms of asthma were the product of 'irritations, however obscure', he divided the condition into four, often indistinguishable, species: the first species was caused by the accumulation of mucus, precipitated by a predisposition to irritability and triggered by a number of exciting factors; the second species, referred to as 'the Dry Asthma', was also caused by irritation, but in this instance by '*Aerial Acrimony*' or '*subtle matter*' conveyed to the lungs; in the third species, paroxysms were initiated by the need to remove irritants from the abdominal viscera; the final species of asthma was the product of habit, which continued to operate after the initial irritation had been removed. In line with this scheme, treatment should focus on persevering with tonics, reducing any tendency to 'morbid irritability', and 'changing ideas of the mind'.[54]

Bree's approach was not without its own inconsistencies and contradictions. While he explained asthma primarily in terms of attempts to remove excess serum and mucus, he failed to clarify the nature or mechanism of the remote causes that predisposed patients to the overproduction of mucus or the effusion of serum. More pertinently, his dismissal of the nervous origins of asthma was immediately criticized by his peers. In 1800, for example, the surgeon George Lipscomb (1773–1846), who had trained in London but who was practising, like Bree, in Birmingham when he wrote his *Observations on the History and Cause of Asthma*, was particularly keen to refute Bree's argument. Lipscomb's professed aim was not to discredit a professional rival, who was apparently unknown to him personally, but to 'elucidate the history of a very prevalent and distressing disease, which has been hitherto but ill explained, and very unsuccessfully treated'.[55]

Lipscomb objected to many features of Bree's account, criticizing his vague terminology, denouncing his over-reliance on ancient authorities, disputing his speculations about the irritating qualities of serum or the morbid state of the pulmonary vessels, and dismissing his classification of asthma into four species. More particularly, however, Lipscomb challenged Bree's argument that post-mortem dissection had not substantiated Cullen's theory of bronchial constriction; the general relaxation of muscles and fibres after death, Lipscomb argued, rendered it '*impossible* to *demonstrate* the existence of spasm on dissection'. Bree's inference that constriction played no part in asthma was therefore flawed. Equally, however, Lipscomb did acknowledge that Cullen's hypothesis also required 'more substantial proofs'.[56]

Lipscomb replaced the theories of Cullen and Bree with speculations of his own. Accepting the primary role of mucus obstructing the air passages, Lipscomb argued that any bronchial effusion must have originated in the arteries of the lungs. However, in asthmatics, the accumulation of serum in the bronchi was not the result of weakened capillaries, as Bree had assumed, but the product of some irritating, acidic, 'acrid matter' in the blood, which induced the rapid pulse and dyspepsia characteristic of early asthma as well as the paradigmatic shortness of breath. Although Lipscomb admitted that the mechanism by which acids produced irritation remained to be elucidated, he nevertheless insisted that the formation of acid in the blood constituted 'the real cause of Asthma': 'If, then, a definition of Asthma be required, I have no objection to call it, *an excessive contraction of the respiratory muscles, excited by the irritation of acid serum effused from the pulmonary vessels into the vesiculæ and bronchia.'*[57]

One of the clinical advantages of this approach, according to Lipscomb, was that it explained not only the symptoms of asthma but also the inefficacy of both ancient and popular modern treatments. Anti-spasmodics, he argued, had become fashionable amongst those 'brought up at the feet of Dr Cullen', but were generally unsuccessful. Similarly, although their use was supported by a long history, fumigations and inhalations of any kind were of no value unless the serum and mucus had first been removed: 'nor do I think it worth while to combat the *visionary* idea of *aerial* medicines being capable of subduing the violence of the paroxysm, before the serous effusion has been expectorated.'[58] Various preparations incorporating vinegar might be beneficial as expectorants during asthma attacks, but their acidic properties rendered their use hazardous at other times. The safest approach to treatment, for Lipscomb, was a combination of expectorants and blood-letting to remove mucus and relieve 'fullness of the vessels' during an attack, followed by bitters, chalybeate waters, and a suitable regimen to reduce acidity and prevent recurrence.

The dispute between Bree and Lipscomb was not easily resolved; arguments about the precise pathology of asthma persisted throughout the nineteenth century. However, Cullen's spasmodic theory gained support from the influential writings of the French clinician and pathologist René Théophile Hyacinthe Laennec (1781–1826), who had been trained in the arts of diagnosis and pathological anatomy by Jean-Nicolas Corvisart (1755–1821), renowned particularly for promoting the use of thoracic percussion (or tapping the chest) as a diagnostic tool. In 1819, Laennec published the results of his research into the value of auscultation of the chest, in which he attempted to correlate the breath sounds heard through his newly invented stethoscope with autopsy findings. Laennec's work was soon translated into English by John Forbes, leading to the widespread adoption of auscultation across Europe and North America.

Laennec's discussion of asthma was extensive. He recognized that the word had often been applied indiscriminately to a variety of types of breathing difficulty, pointing out that few medical terms had been more abused. Echoing the opinions of Corvisart and Léon Louis Rostan (1790–1866), who had performed autopsies on elderly patients with asthma, Laennec suggested that many forms of asthma were in fact the result of diseases of the heart or large vessels, often referred to by subsequent authors as 'cardiac asthma'.[59] In addition, he noted that many cases of 'humid asthma' were examples of chronic catarrh, in line with Cullen's 'dyspnoea catarrhalis', and that many patients with so-called nervous asthma would eventually be shown to have an organic lesion as yet unrecognized. However, he resisted what he regarded as a common practice among physicians and pathologists of denying the existence of 'spasmodic asthma'. In the second edition of his treatise on auscultation, Laennec argued that the existence of 'circular fibres around the bronchial ramifications', which had been demonstrated by the German physician Franz Daniel Reisseissen (1773–1828), made it 'very conceivable that the spasmodic contraction of these fibres may be carried the length of obstructing the air passages to such a degree as to prevent the transmission of air to a great portion of the lungs'.[60] Evidence that patients with both dry and humid asthma exhibited identical respiratory sounds during inspiration and expiration reinforced his belief that respiratory distress in asthmatics was caused not by mucus, but by 'spasm of the bronchia'. Noting that patients with asthma often suffered from a range of other nervous symptoms, Laennec therefore deduced that the condition was fundamentally 'a nervous affection': 'From all these facts and considerations, I think I am entitled to conclude, that the greater number of asthmatic paroxysms, although depending on several causes combined, are chiefly induced by a primary and momentary alteration in the state of nervous influence.'[61]

Equally shrewd and balanced in his approach to treatment, Laennec emphasized the importance of addressing both the nervous and the organic elements of the disease on an individual basis. Expectorants and emetics such as squills and the roots of the flowering plant ipecacuanha, for example, operated by reducing catarrh, while anti-spasmodics, such as opium, belladonna, stramonium, tobacco, hyoscyamus, and coffee, served effectively to counteract any tendency to nervous spasm. In particularly stubborn cases, Laennec advised simply trying one remedy after another, taking care to employ increasing doses of whole, powdered plants or recently prepared extracts. In passing, Laennec also briefly mentioned the use of oxygen therapy, which had been advocated by Thomas Beddoes (1760–1808) and was subsequently promoted by other authors, and discussed the dangers, as well as possible benefits, of electricity or galvanism promoted by the French obstetrician and Professor of Physics and Chemistry Joseph-Aignan Sigaud de Lafond (1730–1810).

During the middle decades of the nineteenth century, Laennec's speculative reflections on the spasmodic theory of asthma were substantiated by various studies in experimental pathology. In 1833, Charles J. B. Williams (1805–89), who had studied Laennec's methods in Paris, demonstrated that the air passages of most animals possessed an 'irritable contractility', which could be triggered by a range of chemical, electrical, or mechanical stimuli. The following decade, both the French anatomist and physiologist François Achille Longet (1811–71) and the German physiologist Alfred Wilhelm Volkmann (1801–77) confirmed that electrical stimulation of the nerves supplying the lungs caused bronchial constriction. Finally, the Swiss histologist and embryologist Rudolph Albert von Kölliker (1817–1905) reiterated Reisseissen's work by establishing the presence of smooth muscle in the bronchi.[62]

There is some evidence to suggest that contemporary theoretical and experimental preoccupations with nervous spasm were translated into everyday clinical practice. In 1836, the author of a letter to the Scottish surgeon John Campbell (1792–1873) explained a patient's asthmatic symptoms in terms of the local irritability of his lungs combined with a systemic nervous irritability:

> After examining Mr Pritchard with much care, I consider his disease to be essentially asthma, mainly dependent on irritability and susceptibility of the bronchial mucous membrane, evinced by his great tendency to become affected by bronchitis. Associated with this, is a considerable degree of general irritability of the nervous system, displayed by flying pains etc.[63]

While the nervous theory of spasmodic asthma certainly gained adherents on both sides of the Atlantic during the early nineteenth century, it would be a mistake to assume that it was uncritically accepted. Many clinicians and pathologists refused to acknowledge that bronchial constriction constituted the most important feature of the condition and continued to emphasize the role of excess secretion of mucus in causing airway obstruction. While some medical authorities contested experimental demonstrations of bronchial spasm, others, such as Ludwig Traube (1818–76), highlighted the presence of mucus in the bronchi and oedema or swelling of the mucous membranes. Support for this position was evident in a discussion at the Medical Society of London in 1840. Addressing the question 'What is the immediate proximate cause of asthma?', the Society's president, Dr Henry Clutterbuck (1767–1856), introduced the case of a 24-year-old man with 'periodical asthma'. The signs pointed to obstruction 'in the ramifications of the bronchia before they terminated in the air cells'. Dismissing the notion that obstruction arose from spasm, Clutterbuck argued that the primary cause was 'a temporary thickening of the mucous membranes of the bronchial tubes from inflammatory action'. Although several members of the audience rejected Clutterbuck's emphasis on inflammation, they agreed that asthmatic patients did exhibit 'an increased and peculiar sensitiveness of the bronchial mucous membranes'.[64]

However, it is apparent that during the middle decades of the nineteenth century the spasmodic theory was becoming more popular. When the discussion on asthma was resumed at the next meeting of the Medical Society of London, for example, some members contradicted Clutterbuck's argument by pointing to the experiments carried out by Williams, which proved that 'the ramifications of the bronchial tubes were contractile, and would therefore be liable to spasm'.[65] Similarly, North American physicians, such as John A. Swett (1808–54), and many European physicians increasingly regarded bronchospasm, sometimes triggered by inflammation, as the primary cause. This approach is particularly evident in the work of the English physician Henry Hyde Salter (1823–71), who, as an asthmatic himself, well recognized 'the sense of impending suffocation, [and] the agonizing struggle for the breath of life' that accompanied an acute asthma attack.[66] Salter trained and practised in London, at King's College and Charing Cross hospitals, and was elected to both the Royal College of Physicians and the Royal Society. His treatise on asthma, first published in 1860 and based on his own experiences as well as on those of his patients, was a remarkable success. Considered a definitive text for many decades, it appeared in an American edition in 1864 and an expanded second British edition in 1868, establishing Salter's reputation as an expert in the field and increasing the flow of patients to his practice.

Salter subscribed to the nervous theory of asthma. Although he accepted that in occasional cases the trigger appeared to be 'essentially humoral', produced by an irritant in the blood, Salter argued that the 'shrill sibilant whistle' and respiratory distress associated with asthma were caused primarily by 'a spastic contraction of the fibre-cells of organic or unstriped muscle, which minute anatomy has demonstrated to exist in the bronchial tubes', rather than by the presence of bronchial catarrh or bronchitis. Drawing on the work of the English physiologist Marshall Hall (1790–1857), Salter suggested that bronchial constriction was the product of 'excito-motory or reflex action', initiated in these cases by 'deleterious material' entering the air passages. Although Salter accepted that asthma attacks could be precipitated by a variety of factors familiar to most authors since Hippocrates, such as environmental conditions, diet, fatigue, emotions, and respiratory illnesses, he also indicted the greater pressures of modern civilization, particularly in relation to the class distribution of asthma: 'the rich might be really more liable to asthma than the poor, from a more irritable nervous organization engendered by the state of hyper-civilization in which we live'.[67]

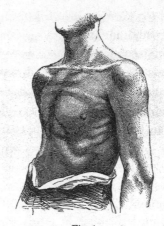

Fig. 4.
From a photograph of an asthmatic, whose disease dated from whooping-cough at three months old.

7. Illustration of an asthmatic from Henry Hyde Salter, *On Asthma* (1860). (*Wellcome Library, London*)

Recognizing the idiosyncratic and familial nature of asthma as well as its close association with hay fever, Salter proposed an account of the condition that prioritized the role of variations in individual sensitivity in determining asthmatic tendencies:

> In what, then, does the peculiarity of the asthmatic essentially consist? Manifestly, in a morbid proclivity of the musculo-nervous system of his bronchial tubes to be thrown into a state of activity; the stimulus may be either immediately or remotely applied, but in either case would not normally be attended by any such result. There is no peculiarity in the stimulus, the air breathed is the same to the asthmatic and non-asthmatic, the ipecacuan powder, the hay effluvium, is the same in both... it is clear that the vice in asthma consists, not in the production of any special irritant, but in the irritability of the part irritated.[68]

Salter's approach to treatment reflected his understanding of the aetiology and pathogenesis of asthma. In alleviating the paroxysms, he emphasized the importance of avoiding or removing any known 'exciting cause', as well as the use of depressants such as ipecacuanha, tobacco, and antimony to suppress nervous irritation, stimulants such as strong black coffee, tea, ammonia, and Indian hemp or *cannabis sativa* to divert 'morbid activity' from the lungs, and sedatives to allay irritability. In a series of articles as well as in his book, Salter described the most effective sedatives in detail, notably tobacco in small doses, chloroform, stramonium, and belladonna, which was being used more frequently both to relieve and to prevent attacks.[69]

Although reviews of his book claimed that Salter had overestimated 'the novelty and originality of many of his leading principles',[70] it does appear that Salter's work marked an important shift in conceptions of asthma. While his focus on nervous bronchial constriction can be clearly traced to earlier Enlightenment formulations of asthma and while many authors had noted the idiosyncratic and capricious nature of asthma, Salter's strong emphasis on a constitutional predisposition to the disease, rather than on precise environmental triggers, marked a critical departure from previous understandings. Salter's ideas were reiterated and refined by other contemporary medical authors, notably by the French physician Armand Trousseau (1801–67), who was renowned both for being the first French doctor to perform a tracheotomy and for his description of how to elicit the neuromuscular excitability characteristic of hypocalcaemia (low blood calcium). According to Trousseau, asthma was often associated with eczema and hives, and the tendency to develop these conditions was inherited in the form of what he termed a 'diathetic neurosis'.[71] Significantly, it was this notion of asthma as part of a constellation of closely related and jointly inherited clinical conditions that came to dominate subsequent accounts and experiences of the disease.

As we have seen, medical and personal accounts of asthma published between the Renaissance and the mid-nineteenth century demonstrate both continuity and change. On the one hand, it would appear that John Floyer, Tobias Smollett, Robert Bree and Henry Hyde Salter suffered from much the same paroxysms of breathlessness, wheezing, and coughing as Seneca and other asthmatics had in previous centuries. Equally, the introduction of a range of novel diagnostic techniques, such as auscultation, percussion, and spirometry (which had been developed in the 1840s by the English surgeon John Hutchinson (1811–61) as a means of measuring lung capacity), combined with new forms of pathological investigation to reinforce traditional beliefs that the lungs were the principal organs involved in asthma. Moreover, modern treatments for asthma often reiterated the advice and prescriptions specified by classical and medieval medical commentators. In 1861, for example, the Devon surgeon Thomas Pridham (1803–73) continued to recommend emetics to remove irritants from the blood and relieve the respiratory distress associated with asthma.[72]

On the other hand, theories and patterns of the disease clearly shifted during this period. Although most writers acknowledged that the causes of asthma were complex and that the accumulation of phlegm or mucus in the lungs might play a part as ancient authors had suggested, there was an emerging consensus that the symptoms of asthma were primarily the product of a constitutional nervous irritability leading to bronchial constriction. In addition, novel environmental and occupational

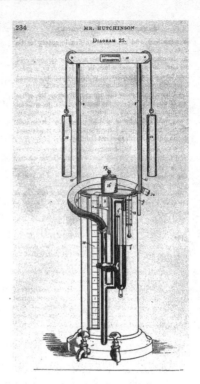

8. John Hutchinson's spirometer, 1846. (*Wellcome Library, London*)

hazards were recognized as triggers of respiratory distress, including asthma: in the 1820s, an outbreak of a fatal inflammatory disease amongst dockyard workers in Plymouth, England, was tentatively linked to exposure to mineral tar, which was regarded by some workers as a treatment for asthma but which was discovered to cause respiratory problems such as coughing and bronchial constriction.[73] At the same time, new remedies for asthma were introduced into the Western therapeutic arsenal. Encouraged by a wave of fashionable 'orientalism' spreading through Europe during the early decades of the nineteenth century, some of these fresh remedies were imported from the East. Hyoscyamus, certainly prescribed from the seventeenth century in England and recommended by Laennec, had been used in the form of henbane by Indian and Egyptian physicians for many centuries. More particularly, the inhalation of preparations of thorn apple or *Datura stramonium*, which possessed similar properties to henbane and which was referred to by one grateful patient as 'the divine Stramonium',[74] was introduced into British medicine in the early nineteenth century by General Gent, who had obtained this indigenous remedy from James Anderson (*c*.1740–1809), the Scottish-born physician-general in Madras. As several medical texts suggest, stramonium rapidly became popular amongst asthmatic patients and their physicians, partly because it reportedly induced 'a grateful forgetfulness and a balmy oblivion like opiates'.[75]

Although there was perhaps greater consensus by the mid-nineteenth century regarding the pathology of asthma, many aspects of the condition remained uncertain. Medical writers continued their attempts to clarify the distribution of asthma according to age, sex, class, and race, to distinguish between genuine spasmodic asthma and what were often regarded as spurious forms of the disease such as thymic or laryngeal asthma, to expose the nature of emergent links with other conditions such as hay fever and eczema, and to elucidate the biological basis of the idiosyncratic or capricious character of the disease. In addition, there were debates about the severity and potential fatality of asthma. During the eighteenth and nineteenth centuries, most physicians believed that asthma was rarely fatal, unless the condition was either caused or complicated by other respiratory or cardiac complaints, such as consumption or an aneurysm. Although contemporary figures rarely distinguished between the various forms of asthma, doctors' case books, hospital records, and official mortality statistics from England do suggest that in some cases asthma could kill. In 1841, for example, the annual national figures provided by the Registrar General suggested that 5,183 people died from asthma; within London, deaths from asthma numbered 355, compared with 1,959 from consumption, 239 from measles, and 254 from smallpox. As several commentators pointed out, mortality statistics suggested that deaths from asthma increased during the autumn and winter and that they were more frequent in towns than in the country, possibly as a result of air pollution. In addition, unlike most respiratory conditions, which were more often fatal in early childhood, deaths from asthma occurred most frequently in patients over the age of 50.[76] Although the potential fatality of asthma continued to be disputed, it is evident that during the late nineteenth and early twentieth centuries new theories of disease and collective health statistics gradually began to challenge individual accounts of asthma as a periodically distressing, but relatively rare and mild, condition.

III

~∞~

ASTHMA, ALLERGY,
AND THE MIND

My attacks come and go without forewarning. I take inhalations every day. The only rest I take is frequently put off
until four or five o'clock in the morning. How can I receive
anyone? Certainly there are some less bad days. I make use
of them by getting up and going out, but I don't know in
advance. I can only be patient and hope.

Marcel Proust, letter to Jean-Louis Vaudoyer, 1912

On 7 December 1889, an American inventor, Frederick
Augustus Roe, obtained a patent for a device that
was designed both to cure and to prevent not only
the deadly strain of influenza that was sweeping across Europe
from Russia, but also a wide range of other respiratory complaints, including catarrh, bronchitis, coughs and colds, croup,
whooping cough, hay fever, and asthma. Sold from offices in
Hanover Square in London for ten shillings, the Carbolic Smoke
Ball comprised a hollow ball of India rubber containing carbolic acid powder. When the ball was compressed, a cloud of
particles was forced through a fine muslin or silk diaphragm
to be inhaled by the consumer. Boosted by testimonials from

satisfied customers and endorsements from prominent doctors, Roe was sufficiently confident that the contraption would
prevent influenza that, in several advertisements placed in the
Illustrated London News and the *Pall Mall Gazette* during the winter
of 1891, he offered to pay £100 to any person who contracted
influenza 'after having used the ball 3 times daily for two weeks
according to the printed directions supplied with each ball'. As
if to demonstrate the sincerity of this offer, Roe claimed to have
deposited £1,000 with the Alliance Bank in Regent Street.

In November 1891, Louisa Elizabeth Carlill, the wife of a law-
yer, purchased a Carbolic Smoke Ball in London and carefully
followed the instructions for use. When Mrs Carlill contracted
influenza the following January, her husband wrote to Roe
claiming the 'reward' offered in the advertisements. Suggesting
that the claim was fraudulent, Roe refused to pay and provided
Mr Carlill with the names of his solicitors. In the resulting legal
case, initially heard in the court of Queen's Bench and subsequently reviewed by the Appeal Court, the dispute did not
revolve primarily around whether the plaintiff had used the
device correctly or indeed whether or not she had contracted
influenza; these issues were largely accepted as fact. Rather,
legal arguments focused on whether the advertisement constituted a valid offer, rather than 'a mere puff', as Lord Justice
Bowen neatly put it, and whether Mrs Carlill's use of the smoke
ball constituted acceptance of that offer. By deciding unani-
mously in Mrs Carlill's favour, the English courts set a precedent
regarding unilateral contracts that continued to inform the legal
doctrines of offer and acceptance, consideration, misrepresen-
tation, and wagering throughout the twentieth century.[1]

While *Carlill v. Carbolic Smoke Ball Company* became a celebrated
moment in legal history, it also reveals several dimensions of

9. Advertisement for the Carbolic Smoke Ball, c.1891. (*Courtesy of the Advertising Archives, London*)

contemporary approaches to respiratory diseases, including asthma. In the first instance, it demonstrates the growing popularity of inhalation as a treatment. Ancient Greek, Egyptian, and Indian doctors had certainly recommended burning and inhaling smoke from a variety of plants to relieve asthma and catarrh, but this therapeutic approach blossomed from the mid-eighteenth century with the invention of several patent inhalers, such as those introduced in the 1760s and 1770s by the English physicians Philip Stern and John Mudge (1721–93). These devices allowed effective delivery of hot vapours from menthol, camphor, eucalyptus, and balsam directly to the lungs. Indeed, according to the author of a short tract entitled *Instant Relief to the Asthmatic*, published in 1774, the inhalation of medications for asthma was greatly superior to 'inward applications', which resulted in the drugs being 'separated and subtilized by the body' before reaching the lungs. In this instance, inhalation of vaporized acid salts, or 'aetherial essence', supposedly operated by loosening phlegm, increasing expectoration, and easing respiration.[2]

During the nineteenth century, a variety of new inhalation devices were introduced across Europe and North America, including the 'bronchitis kettle', the white or marbled glazed earthenware inhalers originally designed by Dr Nelson but produced and improved by Maw and Son from the mid-Victorian period, the 'Vapo-cresolene' vaporizer, and 'Maxim's Pipe of Peace', as well as the notorious Carbolic Smoke Ball. In each case, the apparatus facilitated the inhalation of fumes from a variety of individual antiseptic agents such as carbolic acid, creosote, and chloroform, or from mixtures such as Friar's Balsam. As Marcel Proust's efforts to relieve his own shortness of breath demonstrate, patients could also purchase anti-asthma cigarettes and powders, which usually contained stramonium or potash but sometimes included narcotics. Preparations such as Potter's Asthma Cigarettes, Himrod's Cure for Asthma, Asthmador Cigarettes, Dr J. D. Kellogg's Asthma Remedy, Espic, Legras, and Escouflaire powders, and ozone paper were aggressively marketed and sold over the counter in most Western countries. The popularity of such treatments was documented in contemporary novels. In *David Copperfield*, for example, the asthmatic Charles Dickens (1812–70), whose son represented Mrs Carlill at the appeal, described how the draper, Mr Omer, smoked 'for the asthma'.[3] Although such remedies were sometimes criticized because they were thought to increase bronchial inflammation, by the end of the nineteenth century fumigations, inhalations, and smoking constituted a first line of treatment for many asthmatics.

As the correspondence pages of Victorian medical journals confirm, Mrs Carlill was not alone in desperately seeking a preventative or cure for a respiratory complaint. In 1863, a letter to the *Lancet* from a doctor requested advice from his colleagues about how best to manage regular attacks of 'spasmodic asthma', which had so far resisted any treatment: 'Can it be possible that medicine,' the author concluded, 'which has done so much for other diseases, can do nothing for one of the most distressing complaints that man is heir to?' Over the following weeks, a number of medical practitioners responded by promoting their own preferred forms of treatment.[4] In this period, there were almost as many potential remedies as there were practitioners. Treatment options included not only the familiar array of antispasmodics, expectorants, and dietary advice recommended by Henry Hyde Salter, Armand Trousseau, and other leading medical authorities, but also alcohol, potassium nitrate, potassium

Why Suffer from Asthma?

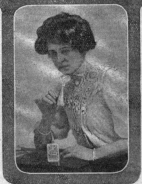

YOU know how exhausting asthma is. You know how prostrated you are by an attack. Year after year you have suffered in this way. The slightest thing brings on the dreaded paroxysms of coughing, and the perpetual fear of an attack coming on, makes life a misery. Not only is the attack painful and prostrating, but the loss of time during your absence from business is another serious item in the account, and that is why you would give anything for a remedy that would afford you prompt and certain relief and freedom from attacks. That is why you ought to know about " Potter's Asthma Cure," because it gives

Relief—Instant Relief

in asthma. The use of " Potter's Asthma Cure" will enable you to breathe freely. The paroxysms of coughing will stop, and ease, comfort, and sweet, soothing relief will be yours. In every trouble of the breathing apparatus " Potter's Asthma Cure " is marvellously successful. In asthma, hay fever, bronchitis, and whooping-cough the relief it affords is truly delightful. It enables those who are racked and tortured by incessant coughing to gain restful and refreshing sleep. And the point is that

It's so easy to use

" Potter's Asthma Cure." You can either put a little of " Potter's Asthma Cure " on a plate and ignite it and inhale the fumes, or you can use " Potter's Patent Inhaler," which is far more convenient, and costs but one shilling. In either case the virtues are brought directly into contact with the breathing organs, and immediately " Potter's Asthma Cure " is used you are conscious of a feeling of soothing, calming relief, which is most grateful. Until you have tried " Potter's Asthma Cure " you cannot realise what it will do for you. Possibly you have tried some other so-called cure and been disappointed. " Potter's Asthma Cure " never disappoints, but

gives ease, comfort, and relief. " Potter's Asthma Cure " is

Almost Magical

in the results it produces, whilst it is at the same time quite safe. It is entirely free from opium, and does not cause headache, as is the case with other so-called remedies. Furthermore, " Potter's Asthma Cure " has no injurious effects on the general health, so that there is no room for hesitation about using it. Why be tortured and prostrated by asthma and its agonies when you can gain sweet and immediate relief by using " Potter's Asthma Cure " ?

Potter's Asthma Smoking Mixture

is purely herbal in its composition, and it may be smoked in a pipe either with or without ordinary tobacco. All that has to be done to prevent the paroxysms of asthma is to draw the smoke well into the lungs and bronchial passages, and relief will immediately be obtained. For asthmatic subjects who are compelled to be out of doors, " Potter's Asthma Smoking Mixture " possesses very great advantages, which we have found have been greatly appreciated by the public.

Potter's Asthma Cure Cigarettes

are in every way as convenient and efficacious as the Smoking Mixture. They enable those whose business calls them out of doors to carry the remedy for their trouble in their pockets with them. At the first symptoms of an attack " Potter's Asthma Cigarettes " should be smoked, and in that way pain, discomfort, and suffering will be avoided. " Potter's Asthma Cigarettes " are specially valuable in foggy weather and on going into the open air, and their use is a wonderful protection. The same thing is true of " Potter's Smoking Mixture." A cigarette smoked by the asthmatic the last thing at night will ensure a good night's rest and pleasant refreshing sleep.

10. Advertisement for Potter's Asthma Cure, c.1910. (*Wellcome Library, London*)

iodide, ether, chloroform, sulphurous baths, arsenic, phosphor-
ous acid, and injections of atropine into the pneumo-gastric
nerve. In some cases, a change of locality or travel abroad to
areas where the air was purer and cleaner were regarded as the
simplest means of engineering immediate relief.

The case of *Carlill v. Carbolic Smoke Ball Company* also suggests
that, as in earlier times, the diagnostic and symptomatic boundaries between respiratory diseases were fairly fluid in this period.
Although the wide range of conditions for which the Carbolic
Smoke Ball was recommended should be understood primarily as a marketing strategy, it is evident that there was indeed
considerable overlap between asthma, bronchitis, emphysema,
tuberculosis, and many other respiratory conditions. The relationship between asthma and other lung diseases had been
regularly explored by medical writers during the early modern
period and in some cases the presence of complications such as
consumption and dropsy was regarded as the principal cause of
mortality in patients with asthma. These associations persisted.
As both contemporary medical writings and the admission of
children to Great Ormond Street Hospital indicate, during the
nineteenth century asthma, emphysema, bronchitis, and consumption continued to be regarded as diseases that not only
shared similar symptoms but also often coexisted in the same
patient. Equally, it was recognized by many medical authors
that the cardinal symptoms associated with asthma since
antiquity, notably cough, wheezing, and respiratory distress,
could also be generated by pathology outside the lungs, giving
rise to conditions that could readily be confused with bronchial asthma, such as cardiac, thymic, and dyspeptic varieties
of asthma. Indeed, early twentieth-century medical textbooks
and dictionaries listed over fifteen types of asthma, including

not only the most common form of bronchial or spasmodic asthma, but also asthma caused by occupational exposure to dusts, reflex asthma, sexual asthma triggered either by venereal disease or excessive excitement, amygdaline asthma caused by enlarged tonsils and adenoids, and asthma nocturnum that was due to nightmares.[5]

However, while these clinical correlations and manifestations continued to be described and disputed in medical journals, a new range of connections was rapidly emerging that would substantially reorient understandings of asthma in the twentieth century. In a letter to the *Lancet* published in 1868, an English doctor noted that 'asthma and eczema are frequently present in the same subject'.[6] Some years later, J. B. Berkart, physician to the City of London Hospital for Diseases of the Chest, confirmed the link in his provocative study of the pathology and treatment of bronchial asthma first published in 1878:

> Various kinds of skin diseases are met with in one-fourth of all cases...Eczema, the most frequent of all, generally dates from earliest infancy, and presents a remarkable chronicity, as well as a great tendency to acute exacerbations. As the eczema passes through its several stages when the dyspnœa has already abated, the theory has been started that there is an alternation between diseases of the skin and the bronchial surface, the implication of the one relieving the other.[7]

At much the same time, clinicians were suggesting similar links between asthma and hay fever, which had first been clearly described by the English physician John Bostock (1773–1846) in 1819. Indeed, cases of respiratory distress seemingly provoked by the same environmental triggers as hay fever were routinely referred to as 'hay asthma'. Increasingly, this clinical triad of asthma, eczema, and hay fever was regarded as a group of closely related conditions, which not only frequently coexisted in the same patient or family but also shared a common set of physical and psychological features.

Allergy and anaphylaxis

In the late nineteenth century, asthma was regarded by most medical commentators as a relatively uncommon condition that was distressing but rarely fatal. According to the British physician Walter Hayle Walsh (1812–92), the deaths recorded from asthma in the Registrar General's annual reports were attributable not primarily to asthma but, as many earlier studies had intimated, to 'a vast number of cases where pulmonary and cardiac disease coexisted'. Significantly, in the revised and enlarged fourth edition of his textbook on diseases of the lungs published in 1871, Walshe went further to suggest that the presence of asthma, much like gout in the eighteenth century, was entirely consistent with long life and that it prevented patients from developing more serious conditions.

> Spasmodic asthma not only does not directly destroy, but is compatible with remarkable prolongation of, life: the popular adage likens the possession of the disease to a 'lease of long life'. The blood-state in asthma is, probably, unfavourable in the main to the occurrence of, and *pro tanto* saves the patient from, various grave diathetic diseases; while the habitual caution, the patient is forced to observe hygienically, saves him from acute inflammatory disorders.[8]

Walshe's views were confirmed by others, most notably the American physician Oliver Wendell Holmes (1809–94), himself an asthmatic, and the Canadian physician and Regius Professor of Medicine at Oxford, William Osler (1849–1919), who insisted that death during an asthma attack was unknown.[9] Although one or two children were certainly admitted to Great Ormond Street Hospital in London each year with a diagnosis of asthma during the second half of the nineteenth century and although some medical writers warned that reliable mortality data were not yet available, surveys of hospital admissions and mortality rates tended to corroborate contemporary beliefs that asthma was infrequent and mild: studies in both Scotland and London in the nineteenth century suggested that less than 0.1 per cent of hospital admissions were for asthma and it would appear that no deaths from asthma occurred at Westminster Hospital between 1884 and 1914.[10]

While most doctors agreed that asthma was extremely unlikely to be fatal unless complicated by other more serious conditions, approaches to the precise pathology of asthma were deeply divided. On the one hand, many physicians continued to support the theory of nervous bronchospasm that had been introduced in the eighteenth century by Cullen and developed by Laennec and Salter in the nineteenth century. According to Walshe, for example, the clinical features of spasmodic asthma were the product of 'tonic contraction of the circular fibres' of the bronchi caused by 'perverted innervation'. The condition could be the result of either a primary neurosis triggered by internal reflex mechanisms, or a secondary neurosis initiated by the local 'irritant influence of bronchitis or emphysema'.[11]

On the other hand, a number of medical authorities continued to insist that bronchospasm was not the only, and perhaps not even the primary, mechanism involved. Instead, they echoed ancient formulations of asthma by highlighting its catarrhal, inflammatory nature. In 1852, the American physician J. A. Swett acknowledged that bronchospasm was important, but regarded 'bronchial inflammation' as the 'principal exciting cause of the paroxysm'.[12] Swett's views were reinforced by opponents of the spasmodic theory, such as Berkart, who not only rejected claims that asthma was the product of 'mysterious derangements of the nervous system', but also insisted that anti-spasmodics had so far failed to furnish asthmatics with significant relief from their distress. Instead, Berkart asserted that respiratory distress in asthma was more likely to be caused by transient obstruction of the bronchi.[13] Similarly, the British homoeopath and general practitioner Charles Harrison Blackley (1820–1900), who first identified pollen as the immediate cause of hay fever in 1873, argued that the symptoms of hay asthma were largely due to inflammation of the 'submucous cellular tissue' of the bronchi rather than 'spasm of the circular muscles of the bronchial tubes'.[14]

A growing emphasis on inflammation and mucous obstruction was partially supported by pathological findings, as gradual adoption of the microscope and new staining techniques provided clearer views of cells and their components. In the 1870s, the German clinician Ernst Victor von Leyden (1832–1910) suggested that the presence of crystals in the sputum, first described by Jean-Martin Charcot (1825–93), might be significant. In particular, von Leyden believed the crystals to be a possible cause of bronchospasm. Some years later, another German physician, Heinrich Curschmann (1846–1910), described spiral structures in the sputum of asthmatic patients and suggested that both spirals and crystals were mucinous plugs that had formed in the smaller airways. The subsequent identification of eosinophils (a type of white blood cell) in both the sputum and the blood of asthmatics in the 1890s, and a demonstrable correlation between the presence of Charcot–Leyden crystals and eosinophils, confirmed speculations that inflammatory exudates played a pivotal role in bronchial asthma.[15]

Although tensions between proponents of the two theories persisted, at the dawn of the twentieth century many writers regarded bronchospasm and mucosal inflammation as parallel and coexistent, rather then mutually exclusive, processes. Thus, the French physician Édouard Brissaud, whose works were well known to Marcel Proust, considered the symptoms of asthma to be the product of both bronchospasm and hypersecretion, which constituted a form of 'bronchial urticaria'. This compromise was elaborated further by Arthur Foxwell (1853–1909), whose career as Professor of Therapeutics at the University of Birmingham was cut short by a tragic bicycle accident. In 1895, Foxwell suggested that attacks of asthma were characterized by a combination of bronchial oedema, bronchial constriction, and contraction of blood vessels in the lungs.[16]

Yet, even as some middle ground was being established between proponents of the spasmodic and mucosal theories of asthma, a novel conceptual framework for understanding the condition was beginning to emerge. In his seminal textbook *The Principles and Practice of Medicine*, first published in 1892 but regularly appearing in revised editions over the next few decades, William Osler reviewed the most prominent contemporary theories of asthma: the popular theory of bronchospasm, which had not been confirmed by experiments according to Osler; suggestions that attacks were due to 'swelling of the bronchial mucous membrane'; the notion that asthma constituted a 'special form of inflammation of the smaller bronchioles—*bronchiolitis exudativa*'; and the possibility that asthma might be caused by reflex spasm of the diaphragm and other respiratory muscles. While he acknowledged that asthma was 'a neurotic affection' and while he did not entirely dismiss alternative theories, Osler suggested that the clinical similarities between hay fever and asthma deserved further attention: 'Making due allowance for anatomical differences, if the structural changes occurring in the nasal mucous membrane during an attack of hay fever were to occur also in various parts of the bronchial mucosa, their presence there would afford a complete and adequate explanation of the facts observed during a paroxysm of bronchial asthma.'[17]

Osler's belief that hay fever and asthma shared the same origins and differed 'only in site' drew heavily on the work of Sir Andrew Clark (1826–93), Emeritus Professor of Clinical Medicine at the London Hospital. According to Clark, although bronchial contraction might occur, it could not be 'the chief factor in the evolution of the asthmatic paroxysm'. Instead, he suggested that asthma, much like hay fever and nettle rash, had 'its roots in a special vulnerability of the respiratory mucous membrane', which responded to irritation by 'hyperaemic swelling' and the secretion of 'a viscid mucus'. Similar views on the close relation between hay fever and asthma were expressed by Charles Blackley and by the celebrated London physician Morell Mackenzie (1837–92), who provided medical endorsements for the Carbolic Smoke Ball in the 1890s and who regarded catarrh and asthma primarily as manifestations of the same underlying predisposition to hay fever.[18]

A burgeoning link between asthma and hay fever was important. By the early twentieth century, hay fever was regarded by many European and North American clinicians as an 'aristocratic disease', more common among the educated, civilized elite than among the lower classes. Portrayed by Clark, and indeed by the American physician George Beard (1839–83), as the product of a 'nervous constitution' exposed to the 'complex influences of over-civilization', hay fever signified intellectual, social, and cultural superiority. 'Sufferers from hay fever may, however, gather some crumbs of comfort', wrote Mackenzie in 1887, 'from the fact that the disease is almost exclusively confined to persons of cultivation'.[19] This image of hay fever and asthma as diseases of luxury and intellectual refinement was both embodied and reinforced in this period, not only by the experiences and examples of prominent creative asthmatics, such as Marcel Proust and the Austrian composers Arnold Schoenberg (1874–1951) and Alban Berg (1885–1935), but also by references in contemporary Western literature. In E. M. Forster's *Howards End*, first published in 1910, hay fever constituted a potent symbol and guardian of innate cultural refinement, distinguishing the upper-class Schlegels from the humble insurance clerk Leonard Bast. Similarly, in 1924, the actor and playwright Noël Coward (1899–1973) employed the term 'hay fever' as the title of a play about upper-class English eccentricity.

At the same time, hay fever and hay asthma were also understood to be the products of an inherited, idiosyncratic susceptibility to pollen, a view that had been independently established in the 1870s both by Blackley in Britain and by Morrill Wyman (1812–1903) in America. The notion of idiosyncrasy was an ancient one that had been discussed occasionally in relation to asthma as well as various adverse reactions to foods and drugs, but clinical interest in the capricious nature of individual vulnerability and in the seemingly unpredictable periodicity of asthma attacks blossomed in the late nineteenth century. At the start of the twentieth century, these notions of excessive sensitivity to foreign agents were effectively reformulated in terms of an overactive or hypersensitive immune system—that is, in terms of anaphylaxis and allergy.

The concept of anaphylaxis was introduced in 1902 by two French physiologists, Charles Richet (1850–1935) and Paul Portier (1866–1962). While attempting to immunize animals against toxins from sea anemones, Richet and Portier noticed that respiratory distress and death sometimes followed a second dose of toxin. Believing the effects to be the result of reduced immunity to the toxin, they termed this phenomenon anaphylaxis, literally meaning the absence of protection. Four years later, an Austrian paediatrician, Clemens von Pirquet (1874–1929), combined these experimental insights with observations from his own studies of serum sickness, carried out with the Hungarian Béla Schick (1877–1967), to develop the notion of allergy. Like Richet and Portier, von Pirquet noted how children immunized against common infectious diseases, such as diphtheria and scarlet fever, in the wards of the Universitäts Kinderklinik in Vienna reacted differently on second exposure to the vaccine. According to von Pirquet, however, the differences were not the result of reduced protection, as Richet and Portier had surmised, but the product of an overactive or supersensitive immune response. Von Pirquet proposed the term 'allergy' to denote this altered reactivity.

Although von Pirquet's suggestion that the body's response, rather than an external pathogen, might be the primary cause of disease was not universally accepted, the clinical implications of his theory were immediately apparent. Indeed, von Pirquet himself emphasized the potential role of allergic reactions in a number of clinical situations: 'Among the allergens should be included the poisons of mosquitoes and bees in so far as their stings are followed by hypo- or hypersensitivity. For this reason we may also enrol under this term the pollen causing hay fever (Wolff–Eisner), the urticaria-producing substances of strawberries and crabs, and probably too a number of organic substances leading to idiosyncrasy.'[20]

It was not long before asthma was included in the list of possible allergic conditions. In 1910, Samuel Meltzer (1851–1920), a leading American physiologist and founder of the Society of Experimental Biology and Medicine, clearly set out the correlation between the clinical features of asthma and those of experimental anaphylaxis. Arguing that explanations focusing on swelling of the mucous membranes or on centrally induced bronchial contraction were not sufficient to account for the symptoms and signs of asthma and noting that atropine not only relieved asthma but also abolished anaphylactic reactions, Meltzer suggested that asthma was essentially the product of anaphylaxis rather than neurosis: 'The theory is here offered that asthma is an anaphylactic phenomenon; that is, that asthmatics are individuals who are "sensitized" to a specific substance and the attack of asthma sets in whenever they are "intoxicated" by that substance.'[21]

The closely associated concepts of allergy and anaphylaxis did not immediately transform clinical understandings, or indeed patient experiences, of asthma, which was still regarded by many commentators primarily as a form of neurosis. However, the reflections of Richet and von Pirquet encouraged further clinical and laboratory research into the precise mechanisms involved in asthma and ultimately laid the foundations for new forms of treatment. Motivated by reports of rising levels of asthma and other allergic conditions particularly in the Western world, during the 1910s, 1920s, and 1930s researchers on both sides of the Atlantic, many of whom were, like their predecessors, asthmatic or allergic themselves, began to explore the cardinal clinical and epidemiological characteristics of asthma and its relation to other allergic diseases in more detail. In many cases, such research served largely to refine and reframe, rather than refute, traditional ancient, medieval and early modern notions of asthma.

In 1916, two leading American allergists from New York, Robert A. Cooke (1880–1960) and Albert Vander Veer (1880–1959), published the results of a study into the pattern of inheritance of allergic diseases, including asthma, hay fever, urticaria, and food sensitivities, in over 500 patients. The notion that asthma was familial and linked to other conditions was not new, having been recognized and discussed by many medical authorities, including Joan Baptista van Helmont, William Cullen, and Henry Hyde Salter. The results of Cooke and Vander Veer's work confirmed that the broad tendency to exhibit allergies was inherited and led to speculations that the expression of allergic diseases was determined by the inheritance of a dominant characteristic. In subsequent studies, in which Cooke and Arthur F. Coca (1875–1959) attempted to classify immunological hypersensitivity more precisely, this familial tendency to suffer from allergy was referred to as 'atopy', derived from Greek and meaning literally 'out of place'. Increasingly, in most medical accounts the terms 'allergy', 'atopy', and 'anaphylaxis' were used interchangeably to describe the collection of diseases generated by immunological hypersensitivity.[22]

Research into the mechanisms of allergic reactions also furnished new insights into the pathogenesis of asthma and other conditions, leading ultimately to new pharmacological approaches to the treatment of asthma, hay fever, and food allergies. Experimenting on themselves at the Institute of Hygiene in Breslau, in 1921 Carl Prausnitz (1876–1963) and Heinz Küstner

(1897–1963) demonstrated that sensitivity to fish could be transferred passively from one subject to another with serum. These results suggested that certain allergic reactions were mediated by specific antibodies, as von Pirquet had radically suggested in his earlier studies of vaccination reactions. The antibody responsible for what became known as the Prausnitz–Küstner reaction, and indeed for other manifestations of allergy, was increasingly referred to as 'reagin' or 'reaginic antibody'.[23]

The concepts of atopy and antibody-mediated allergic sensitivity certainly clarified and consolidated clinical understandings of asthma and related conditions. However, questions remained about the manner in which asthmatic patients were sensitized, about the precise nature of the sensitizing substances, and about how best to demonstrate and evaluate sensitivity in the clinic. In particular, skin tests for allergic sensitivity, introduced by the American allergist Isaac Chandler Walker (1883–1950), proved problematic, since they were often negative in asthma patients. Reviewing Walker's reflections on the causes of bronchial asthma in 1922, Robert Cooke insisted that Walker's notion of 'intrinsic' bacterial sensitization was unproven and refuted his argument that substances such as hay dust and house dust operated as non-specific irritants of the respiratory mucous membranes. For many centuries, dust had been recognized and feared as a potent trigger of asthma attacks and had led directly to production of the first electric vacuum cleaner in 1908: the novel suction machine, initially invented and patented that year by an asthmatic American janitor, James Murray Spangler (1848–1915), in order to reduce his exposure to dust at work, was subsequently manufactured and distributed by William H. Hoover (1849–1932). According to Cooke, who was himself asthmatic, various dusts in the home and workplace operated not as mechanical irritants, as some physicians had assumed, but as 'genuinely specific factors' or allergens: 'These cases indicate that attacks of asthma on exposure to dusty hay are not to be considered as a reflex effect of a non-specific excitant, as Walker states, but as an expression of a specific allergic reaction.'[24]

Although alternative explanations of asthma persisted, these seminal studies carried out largely by American and German clinicians firmly established asthma as 'the chief clinical manifestation of the hypersensitive state [or allergy] in human beings'.[25] While early attention had centred largely on hay fever as the archetypal allergic disorder, during the middle decades of the twentieth century asthma increasingly became the most prominent focus for specialists in the new field of allergy. Rising interest in exploring the pathological processes and more effectively alleviating the symptoms of asthma generated new clinical initiatives, most notably the creation of laboratories and clinics dedicated to furthering medical knowledge of the mechanisms involved in asthma attacks and to treating asthma and allergy patients. Part of a wider trend towards the establishment of scientific laboratories within hospitals in this period, allergy and asthma clinics appeared first in the United States and Britain, where levels of asthma and hay fever were thought to be highest, but also spread throughout Europe and Australasia and some developing countries, such as India, where asthma was also beginning to emerge as a clinical problem.

Clinical studies of asthma

As regular letters to his family and friends make clear, during the 1900s and 1910s Marcel Proust struggled to control his asthma and hay fever effectively, particularly following the death of his mother in 1905. The treatments available to Proust and his contemporaries included not only symptomatic relief with inhaled anti-spasmodics and various stimulants and relaxants but also the careful avoidance of triggers, achieved either by manipulating the domestic environment or by retreating to the mountains or coastal areas where the air was supposedly free from pollen and dust. During the late nineteenth century, the popularity of 'climate therapy' for hay fever and asthma had profitably established certain towns and regions as fashionable health resorts. On the advice of his doctors, for example, Proust periodically travelled to Thonon or Evian-les-Bains on the southern shores of Lake Geneva to relief his asthma and in December 1905 spent six weeks in a sanatorium on the outskirts of Paris. In 1932, Arnold Schoenberg moved from Berlin to Barcelona partly to improve his asthma; two years later, after emigrating to North America, he again relocated from Boston to Los Angeles in search of cleaner, warmer air. Schoenberg was not alone; for several decades around the turn of the nineteenth into the twentieth century, many wealthy American sufferers from hay fever and asthma flocked to luxurious resorts in the White Mountains or Adirondacks to relieve their respiratory distress.[26]

Climate therapy was predicated upon an assumption that hay fever and asthma were caused by exposure either to a toxin in pollen and dust or in some cases to an asthma germ. Supported by influential germ theories of disease as well as by evidence of bronchial inflammation in asthma, it was this latter notion that had generated commercial opportunities for the manufacturers of devices such as the Carbolic Smoke Ball and other inhaled antiseptic agents. Although such interpretations of the direct role of pollen and bacterial toxins were challenged and ultimately rejected by proponents of the allergic theory of disease, these views did encourage the development of a new mode of treatment for asthma and hay fever. In 1903, William P. Dunbar (1863–1922), Director of the State Hygienic Institute in Hamburg, attempted to immunize hay-fever patients passively using a specific antiserum marketed as 'Pollantin'. Believing that Dunbar's technique was both difficult and unlikely to afford much relief and drawing on parallel studies of active vaccination against infectious diseases, two British bacteriologists working in Sir Almroth Wright's Inoculation Department at St Mary's Hospital in London, John Freeman (1876–1962) and Leonard Noon (1877–1913), attempted to induce active immunity by inoculating patients with increasing doses of pollen. First reported in the *Lancet* in 1911, the results of carefully monitored desensitization or allergen immunotherapy, as it became known, were remarkable: the sensitivity of hay-fever patients to pollen could apparently be reduced one-hundredfold.[27]

Over subsequent years, Freeman amended the protocol for desensitization to suit the hectic lifestyles of his predominantly middle-class patients and engineered a lucrative contract with an American pharmaceutical firm, Parke, Davis & Company, to market and distribute commercial 'hay fever reaction outfits'. In addition, Freeman suggested the possibility of extending the process to include asthma and other allergic disorders. It was possible to vaccinate against asthma, he argued, by using preparations of grass pollen for hay asthma, bacterial vaccines for asthma associated with bronchitis, and extracts of dust and animal danders to treat asthma triggered by exposure to horses, cats, dogs, and house dust. This approach to hay fever and asthma proved immediately attractive to clinicians on both sides of the Atlantic who were struggling to provide effective cures for their asthmatic patients. The leading proponents of desensitization in North America were Robert Cooke in New York and Karl Koessler (1880–1925) in Chicago. By providing an alternative to climate therapy and the wide range of patent medicines available over the counter, desensitization rapidly became the cornerstone of treatment for many allergic disorders until well after the Second World War.[28]

The popularity and availability of desensitization for asthma and hay fever were facilitated by the growth of dedicated allergy and asthma clinics on both sides of the Atlantic. The first and almost certainly the largest clinic for many years was run by John Freeman at St Mary's Hospital in London. During the first half of the twentieth century, the Clinic for Allergic Diseases at St Mary's expanded rapidly, becoming an internationally renowned centre of excellence: by the early 1950s, Freeman and his colleagues were not only treating several thousand patients with asthma and hay fever each year, but also conducting research into the mechanisms of allergies and into the efficacy and safety of new treatments. As clinical interest in asthma and other allergies rose in Britain during the inter-war years, other clinics were established throughout the country. Often based in hospitals and dedicated to exploring the distribution, manifestations, and treatment of asthma in particular, allergy clinics and laboratories were opened in Manchester, Liverpool, Edinburgh, Glasgow, Birmingham, Belfast, and London.

These British clinical and scientific initiatives were strongly supported by the establishment of the Asthma Research Council, which had been founded in 1927 by a group of asthma sufferers, including prominent clinicians, scientists, and philanthropists. The first president was Lord Limerick, who 'had been imprisoned by asthma' for more than five years and who was forced to miss the founding meeting of the Council because of an asthma attack.[29] Endorsed by the government and co-ordinated by a medical advisory committee that included John Freeman, Sir Humphry Rolleston (1862–1944), and Sir Arthur Hurst (1879–1944), the Council aimed to promote research into the prevalence, causes, and treatment of asthma and to improve the lives of an estimated 200,000 British asthmatics. As the Minister of Health pointed out in a letter to the Council in 1929, clearer understandings of asthma-related morbidity and mortality and improved methods of prevention and treatment were sorely needed.

> There are no reliable statistics available as to the incidence of asthma. Comparatively few deaths are directly attributable to this disease, and the mortality returns give no indication of the widespread suffering which it causes. There is, however, no doubt that an appreciable proportion of the population is affected by this obscure malady, and that much suffering and unemployment result.[30]

In North America, parallel initiatives led to the foundation of allergy clinics as well as regional and national organizations aimed at promoting research into asthma and related conditions. Clinics were opened by Walker in Boston in 1916 and by Cooke in New York two years later. As in Britain, the growth of asthma and allergy clinics was supported and encouraged by professional societies: the Western Society for the Study of Hay Fever, Asthma and Allergic Diseases, founded in 1923; and the Society for the Study of Asthma and Allied Conditions, established in 1925 by prominent East-coast allergists such as Robert Cooke and Francis M. Rackemann (1887–1973). In 1943, the two societies merged to form the American Academy of

Allergy, dedicated not only to funding research into the causes and mechanisms of asthma and associated conditions, but also to training young doctors in the field. New research was promoted and coordinated by an Allergy Research Council and disseminated through the *Journal of Allergy*, first published in 1929.[31]

While British and American allergists constituted the early pioneers in creating professional networks committed to unravelling the pathology and mitigating the personal impact of asthma, clinical and public interest also emerged in other developed countries during the middle decades of the twentieth century. In mainland Europe, rising trends in asthma and hay fever, combined with the impetus to research provided by the notions of allergy and anaphylaxis, prompted clinicians to establish allergy clinics, instigate clinical training schemes, and publish new journals dedicated to the field. Equally in Australia, clinical interest in asthma rose in the inter-war years and was bolstered in the 1950s and 1960s by the emergence of regional and national asthma foundations largely energized and coordinated by patients and their families. The Asthma Foundation of New South Wales, for example, was made possible by the crusading zeal of Mickie Halliday and Leila Schmidt. Both mothers of asthmatic children, Halliday and Schmidt refused to accept contemporary dismissals of asthmatics as neurotic and campaigned to raise funds for research and to promote public and clinical awareness. Responsible for many therapeutic innovations, such as the asthma swimming programme, members of the Foundation contributed substantially to reframing medical understandings of the condition and to generating support for global initiatives against asthma.[32]

Although allergies were increasingly regarded largely as the product of Western civilized lifestyles, the problems of asthma were clearly not confined to the developed world. As regular contributions to the *Indian Medical Gazette* during the 1920s and 1930s testify, Indian doctors and their patients were as frustrated as their Western counterparts by their inability effectively to prevent or to cure asthma. In 1926, for example, M. A. Krishna Iyer, a physician working in Alipuram Jail in Bellary in southern India, highlighted the problems posed by asthma: 'Few medical men have successfully treated and cured a real case of asthma. The truth of this remark is borne out by the very many and very varied lines of treatment in vogue...We have to-day no rational, standardised and single mode of treatment for asthma.'[33]

Over subsequent decades, Indian medical practitioners attempted to improve clinical diagnosis and management in various ways. In his brief discussion of predisposing factors, Krishna Iyer himself pointed out the importance of recognizing the central role played by 'climatic seasons, food, different occupations or commodities', and emphasized the value of avoiding known triggers. A Calcutta physician, G. Raghunatha Rao, reinforced Krishna Iyer's advice by alerting readers to the features of 'cotton asthma' prevalent in the Madras Presidency cotton-growing areas. In Rao's experience, conventional medical approaches, including the subcutaneous or intramuscular administration of adrenaline, routinely failed; the only effective solution was for his patients to leave their jobs, a remedy that compounded their physical distress with the prospect of poverty.[34]

In addition, clinicians in India highlighted the diagnostic fluidity of the term by revealing the potential differences between Western and Eastern forms of asthma. On the basis of pathological analysis of the level and maturity of eosinophils in the blood and sputum, measured in particular by the Arneth count or index first introduced in 1903, it appeared that asthma in India was much less often allergic than American and British accounts were suggesting. According to studies published in the 1930s, for example, many more cases of asthma in India were secondary to bacterial infections of the respiratory tract. In addition, it became evident that allergic cases were more common in European settlers in India than amongst Indians themselves, not only reinforcing beliefs in the 'rarity of asthma of allergic origin amongst Indians', but also suggesting crucial racial differences in the inheritance and expression of allergic sensitivity.[35] The heterogeneity of presentations and pathological findings in Indian populations reminded researchers that, as in antiquity, asthma constituted a set of symptoms rather than a single, and constant, identifiable disease.

As clinical studies from America, Europe, and India demonstrate, during the inter-war years many features of asthma remained poorly understood, and, apart from the introduction of desensitization, treatment rested largely on the same range of symptomatic remedies that had been available during the nineteenth century. However, the expansion of both medical and public interest in asthma and the creation of dedicated research centres and organizations across the world provided allergists, paediatricians, and respiratory physicians with opportunities to study increasing numbers of patients and to develop clearer models of distribution and inheritance. As a result, new clinical and statistical approaches to the epidemiology, pathogenesis, and treatment of asthma began to emerge, leading ultimately to dramatic changes in the management and prognosis of the condition.

Research conducted between the wars suggested that the relatively benign image of asthma embraced by Osler and others was becoming increasingly untenable. In 1916, Cooke and Vander Veer had estimated that approximately 7 per cent of the American population suffered from allergies. From a study of families in New York in the 1920s, W. C. Spain and Cooke concluded that approximately 3.5 per cent had hay fever or asthma, a figure broadly confirmed by skin tests. Subsequent studies suggested that these figures were rising. In the early 1930s, a number of surveys revealed that over 10 per cent of the American population exhibited clinical features of asthma, eczema, or hay fever, and in 1939 W. C. Service identified asthma alone in 3.6 per cent of people in Colorado Springs. By the early 1940s, Warren T. Vaughan (1893–1944), one of the leading allergists in North America and a relentless popularizer of allergy, warned that the number of asthmatics in the United States was beginning to constitute a major clinical burden. 'Estimates as to the number of asthmatics in the United States', he suggested in typically sensationalist tones, 'range from 600,000 to 3,500,000. Visualize Boston or Chicago with everyone huffing and puffing.'[36]

Although similar figures are not readily available for other regions of the world, some studies suggest that rising admissions to hospital for asthma in Britain paralleled the pattern of morbidity in the United States during the inter-war period. At the same time, there were suggestions that asthma was becoming more serious, with sporadic reports of deaths from asthmatic attacks. While asthma had been uncommon amongst men enlisted in the United States Army during the First World War, largely because most asthmatics would have been excluded from service by the draft-examining boards, some soldiers did suffer from asthma and a proportion of those died: 'Of the 7,445 asthmatics in the army who became sick enough to require hospitalization,' wrote Vaughan in 1934, '35 died and 2,872 were discharged on account of their disability'.[37] In addition, articles published in the medical press, not only in Britain and the United States but also in India, reinforced nascent concerns that asthma could occasionally kill:

> We are going along on a rather smooth sea in believing that deaths from asthma are comparatively rare, and may be if we all come out of the woods, we will find that the number is sufficiently alarming to make us a little more aware of the possibility of death in these cases, and not be so sanguine in our conversation with members of the family.[38]

Accurate estimates of the prevalence and incidence of asthma, and geographical comparisons across time, were hampered by uncertainty about the definition of the condition. In a monumental textbook on asthma and hay fever co-authored with Arthur Coca and August A. Thommen in 1931, Matthew Walzer, chief of the allergy clinic at the Jewish Hospital of Brooklyn and later president of the Society for the Study of Asthma and Allied Conditions, exposed the semantic and clinical difficulties inherent in the field:

> Were the etiology and mechanism of bronchial asthma clearly understood and generally agreed upon, a definition of this condition would be a comparatively simple matter. Unfortunately, a review of the history and theories of the subject reveals a marked diversity of opinion on these questions. Definitions of asthma are consequently as numerous as the theoretical conceptions of it. It is defined as a 'neurosis', 'diathesis', 'inflammation', 'muscular irritability', etc., or as a dyspnea caused by bronchial 'stenosis', 'spasm', 'edema', or 'inflammation', etc.; by pulmonary 'catarrh', 'rigidity', or

'paralysis'; by diaphragmatic spasm; by alkalosis; by hemo-
clastic shock; by anaphylactic shock, etc., *ad infinitum*. The
very multiplicity of definitions emphasizes their inadequacy.
Consequently, the term asthma today has no universally recognized meaning or application.[39]

Other writers were not as discouraging as Walzer. While
Francis Rackemann did accept that it was best to regard the
term 'asthma' primarily 'as denoting a symptom and to think of
"asthma" as in the same category with "headache" or "nausea"
or even "angina"', he nevertheless insisted that 'the symptom
complex which "asthma" represents is so characteristic that
for present convenience it can almost be regarded as a disease
entity, despite the fact that this complex can be produced by
such a wide variety of different causes'.[40]

It was largely Rackemann's more traditional and pragmatic
vision of asthma as clinically distinct, if pathologically obscure,
that drove research into the causes and mechanisms of asthma
during the inter-war years. Thus, although Walzer and others
warned against explaining asthma solely in terms of hypersensitivity, a number of pivotal studies focused precisely on
clarifying links between laboratory models of anaphylaxis
and the clinical features of asthma. In a number of investigations carried out during the 1910s and 1920s, the Nobel Prize-
winning British physiologist and pharmacologist Henry Dale
(1875–1968) and his co-workers at the Wellcome Physiological
Research Laboratories demonstrated that the interaction of
allergens with tissue-fixed antibodies released histamine, a
chemical mediator that was capable of producing many of
the symptoms of anaphylaxis including respiratory distress.
Later studies revealed the role of mast cell degranulation in the
release of histamine and other inflammatory mediators during

allergic reactions. Such research provided a critical framework for developing and evaluating new treatments for hay fever and asthma, most notably early antihistamines such as Torantil, first marketed in the 1920s, and anti-inflammatory agents such as the corticosteroids.[41]

Recognizing that not all asthma could be explained in terms of allergy to external environmental factors, Francis Rackemann also attempted to classify asthma more carefully according to the nature of the trigger and the putative mechanisms. Echoing Walshe's earlier formulation of asthma as either a primary or a secondary neurosis and based on an initial study of 150 asthmatics and a subsequent survey of 1,074 patients, Rackemann divided asthma broadly into two major groups that, although contested, came to dominate theoretical approaches to the condition: wheezing, coughing, and respiratory distress triggered by identifiable external agents, including pollen, dust, food, animal danders, and medicines such as aspirin, and often relieved by altering the environment, were referred to as 'extrinsic' asthma; asthma generated by internal processes such as bacterial infections, chronic bronchitis, emphysema, and other reflex causes was known as 'intrinsic' asthma. A third miscellaneous group comprised patients whose asthma was either unclassified or distinctive in some way, including chronic severe asthma, fatal asthma, which was supposedly more common 'among middle aged women who tend to slight obesity', and asthma with tuberculosis.[42]

Such large-scale studies revealed critical epidemiological features of asthma as it presented in European and North American populations in the early twentieth century. In particular, it became apparent that extrinsic asthma was more common than intrinsic asthma in children and young adults, but that that distribution was reversed with age; indeed, according to Rackemann, extrinsic asthma rarely began after the age of 45. At the same time, surveys suggested that a positive family history and positive skin tests were far more common in extrinsic than intrinsic asthma and that, although men and women appeared to be affected in roughly equal proportions overall, asthma in children under the age of 5 was more common in boys than in girls.[43]

In the process of clarifying the epidemiological distribution and pathological mechanisms of asthma, clinical and laboratory research during the inter-war years also served to undermine earlier images of asthma as a fashionable nervous condition compatible with long life. Although the precise definition of asthma remained contested and although belief in the elite personalities of both asthma and hay fever certainly persisted, the work of Rackemann and others, as well as reports of asthma in the developing world, clearly challenged notions of asthma as an exclusive condition confined to the white, male upper classes, as Morell Mackenzie and his contemporaries had intimated towards the end of the nineteenth century. Increasingly, asthma constituted a disease, or perhaps more accurately a constellation of symptoms, that could afflict anyone regardless of sex, class, age, or race.

The rising trends in asthma revealed by clinical studies during the early twentieth century offered a lucrative market for a blossoming pharmaceutical industry. Chemists, druggists, and small pharmaceutical firms had been producing medicines and inhalation devices for the relief of asthma throughout the nineteenth century. In the early decades of the twentieth century, American companies such as Parke, Davis & Company, H. K. Mulford Company, and the Lederle and

Abbott Laboratories also began to support the production and distribution of extracts of pollen and other allergens for use in skin testing and desensitization therapy. New understandings of the intercellular mechanisms and inflammatory process involved particularly in allergic asthma stimulated both commercial pharmaceutical and state interest in developing, testing, and improving novel anti-asthma drugs, notably anti-cholinergic and adrenergic agents, the methyl xanthines, steroids, and antihistamines.

For many centuries, plants such as thorn apple, henbane, belladonna, and lobelia had been standard treatments for asthma and a number of other respiratory disorders in both Western and Eastern cultures, largely because of their perceived ability both to sedate and to diminish bronchial irritability. During the nineteenth century, the active components of these plants, which were traditionally administered either by inhalation or as a tincture, were identified and increasingly prescribed in their isolated forms. For example, atropine was originally derived from belladonna in 1833, and its ability to block vagal stimulation of the heart was demonstrated in 1867. In the early years of the twentieth century, its anti-cholinergic properties made atropine a popular treatment for asthma until the emergence of superior alternatives with fewer side effects served to undermine its clinical use. Nevertheless, endorsed by physicians, stramonium cigarettes containing atropine continued to be advertised and consumed on both sides of the Atlantic until the 1980s, when growing concerns about the manner in which young people were inhaling or ingesting the cigarettes for their hallucinogenic properties led to their eventual disappearance from the market.[44]

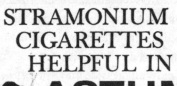

STRAMONIUM CIGARETTES HELPFUL IN ASTHMA

as reported in the British Medical Journal, August 15, 1959

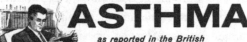

Noted allergist reinvestigates an old treatment for bronchial asthma

For about 150 years Europeans have inhaled smoke from burning stramonium leaves to relieve asthmatic attacks.

Now a noted allergist reports in the British Medical Journal that results of controlled studies leave no doubt that inhaling stramonium (atropine*) smoke has a beneficial effect on the function of the lungs in bronchial obstruction.

The results indicate that smoking stramonium cigarettes has a definite place in the treatment of asthma, increasing the vital capacity and giving a feeling of relief, without unpleasant side effects. In many cases during the controlled study the patients voluntarily commented on their increased ease of breathing.

Stramonium cigarettes have been manufactured by R. Schiffmann Co. for more than 80 years and have been *available without prescription in every drug store* throughout the U. S. and Canada under the name of ASTHMADOR. These cigarettes contain no tobacco and are not habit forming.

ASTHMADOR is also sold in pipe mixture or as aromatic incense powder. Sufferers from bronchial asthma will almost invariably find relief, as indicated in this report.

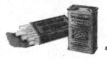

*Atropine is the alkaloid of stramonium.

11. An American magazine advertisement for stramonium cigarettes, *c.*1959. (*Courtesy of the Advertising Archives, London*)

New treatments for asthma were also derived either from plants or from human hormones during the late nineteenth and early twentieth centuries. Since antiquity, Chinese physicians and their patients had used *ma huang,* derived from a shrub commonly found in northern China, to relieve asthmatic parox-ysms. In 1885, the Japanese chemist and pharmacologist Nagai Nagayoshi (1844–1929) successfully isolated an alkaloid from the plant and named it ephedrine, from which he also later synthe-sized methamphetamine. Evidence of ephedrine's physiological actions was provided by studies into the Chinese pharmacopoeia carried out at the Peking Union Medical College in the 1920s by Carl F. Schmidt (1893–1988) and K. K. Chen (1898–1988), who demonstrated the ability of ephedrine to stimulate the heart, promote vasoconstriction, and relax bronchial smooth muscle.

First marketed by Eli Lilly in 1926 and endorsed by clinical trials coordinated by the Medical Research Council during the 1930s, oral and inhaled ephedrine constituted a popular pre-scribed treatment for respiratory conditions for many years. In his autobiography, published in 2008, the novelist and journal-ist Ferdinand Mount (b. 1939) recalled his own reliance on ephe-drine to relieve acute episodes of asthma during his childhood:

> When I have a bad asthma attack, about once a week at this period, he comes over from Warminster without a murmur. Together we go through the motions, I hitch up my pyjama jacket, he listens to my chest, depresses my tongue with the little wooden spatula before peering down my throat and then into my ears. All this I regard as merely the formal pre-liminaries before the real business of handing over the box of little yellow ephedrine pills—half a pill under the tongue magically soothes the tubes, nothing else works, certainly not the breathing exercises the nurses are always teaching me.[45]

In addition, ephedrine was often incorporated into remedies sold over the counter for asthma, hay fever, colds, and bronchi-tis, such as Franol or Franol Plus, which combined ephedrine with theophylline, an antihistamine, and a barbiturate and which was distributed by the Bayer Products Company well into the 1960s. As the radio commentator Tim Brookes recounts in a detailed exploration of his own asthma, although such cocktails of anti-asthma remedies could mitigate the severity of an asthma attack, they often caused intolerable side effects:

> At first, my body started to feel heavy as the phenobarbital kicked in: my limbs felt abandoned, like stuffed bolsters of flesh lying here and there around me—but at the same time my pulse began to pick up and my mind started to race... I would lie there for four or five hours, waiting for the drug to be filtered out of my bloodstream, dragging myself out of bed every couple of hours to take a leak, as Franol also acted as a diuretic. The following morning I was a wreck.[46]

Prior to the marketing of ephedrine, growing pharmaceutical interest in synthesizing active compounds from hormones had already generated drugs capable of directly stimulating the sympathetic nervous system (referred to as sympathomimetic or adrenergic agents) and in the process relieving bronchial obstruction. In 1900, Solomon Solis-Cohen (1857–1948), a clinical lecturer in medicine at Jefferson Medical College in Philadelphia, demonstrated the efficacy of crude adrenal extracts in asthmatic patients. The active substance, known as adrenaline or epinephrine, was successfully isolated and purified by a Japanese chemist, Jokichi Takamine (1854–1922), in 1901. When Jesse G. M. Bullowa and David M. Kaplan from the Montefiore Home for Chronic Invalids in New York reported two years later that hypodermic injections of adrenaline were 'capable of cutting short attacks of asthma', they also contributed to long-standing debates about the pathogenesis of asthma. The efficacy of adrenaline, they suggested, supported arguments that asthma was caused not primarily by bronchospasm but by 'turgidity of the bronchial mucosa'; adrenaline was thought to relieve obstruction by constricting mucosal blood vessels.[47]

Over subsequent decades, adrenaline became one of the first-line treatments for severe asthma in particular. It was administered subcutaneously, intravenously, or in vaporized form by inhalation and was often used in conjunction with other active preparations, including atropine. Significantly, however, modified forms of both ephedrine and adrenaline subsequently replaced the parent compounds in popularity, largely because they acted more selectively on the lungs and therefore caused fewer adverse cardiovascular reactions. Isopropyl adrenaline, or isoproterenol, was introduced in 1903, and isoprenaline was marketed shortly after the Second World War. Although these preparations still carried the risk of cardiac effects, they were more selective than adrenaline and ephedrine and were regularly prescribed in many Western countries throughout the 1940s, 1950s, and 1960s. The careful scientific distinction first between α and β adrenergic receptors in 1948, and subsequently between β_1 receptors in the heart and β_2 receptors in the lungs in 1967, eventually facilitated the development of more specific bronchodilators with minimal cardiac effects, such as salbutamol.[48]

American and German researchers deliberately targeted and exploited other popular remedies for asthma in order to develop more active drugs during the inter-war years. Although not universally accepted, coffee had often been advocated as an effective stimulant and anti-spasmodic since the eighteenth century. In the early 1920s, pharmacological studies at Johns Hopkins University demonstrated the ability of caffeine and other xanthine derivatives, such as theophylline, to relax bronchial muscles and dilate the bronchi. The results of this work, together with parallel studies on theophylline carried out by Samson Hirsch in Frankfurt, were largely ignored by clinicians until the mid-1930s, when a number of anecdotal articles suggested that both theophylline and aminophylline were effective in treating asthma attacks, particularly those resistant to other modes of treatment. The solubility of aminophylline, which had been produced in 1908, made it more suitable for intravenous injection, and it rapidly emerged as a pivotal treatment for patients with adrenaline-resistant 'status asthmaticus', an acute, progressively worsening, and sometimes fatal form of asthma attack.[49]

Significantly, the efficacy of methyl xanthines indirectly supported spasmodic theories of asthma. However, novel remedies also emerged from attempts to alleviate the inflammatory component of bronchial obstruction. Extracts from the adrenal cortex were first used to treat asthma in the 1930s, but the results were equivocal. By the 1940s, however, American reports of the effectiveness of both synthetic cortisone and adreno-corticotrophic hormone (ACTH) in moderating inflammation in patients with rheumatoid arthritis encouraged pharmaceutical companies to test those substances in asthmatics. During the 1950s, controlled trials carried out by the Medical Research Council in Britain, as well as ongoing studies in America, demonstrated the value of oral and intramuscular cortisone in both acute and chronic asthma and indeed in other allergic diseases. Although the adverse effects associated with long-term use of systemic steroids limited their clinical application, they also encouraged the subsequent synthesis of locally active compounds, such as hydrocortisone, for direct delivery to the lungs in asthma or the skin in eczema.[50]

During the middle decades of the twentieth century, some researchers also considered the value of antihistamines for patients with asthma. The discovery of the role of histamine in anaphylactic and allergic reactions had generated interest in developing substances that could block the action of histamine and moderate the symptoms of hay fever and other allergies. During the 1920s and 1930s, a number of antihistamines were developed, and by the 1940s several major European pharmaceutical companies, such as Rhône-Poulenc and Bayer, were actively marketing these preparations for the treatment of allergic diseases. However, in spite of initial optimism on the part of both allergists and the pharmaceutical industry and in spite of evidence that drugs such as chlorpheniramine were effective in hay fever, early clinical trials suggested that antihistamines were of limited value in asthma.[51]

The development of pharmacological approaches to the management of symptoms, and their promotion by a rapidly expanding pharmaceutical industry, clearly changed the prospects for many patients with asthma. However, the wide availability of new treatments did not preclude doctors from devising and promoting their own, sometimes eponymous, therapies. Believing asthma to be a 'vasomotor neurosis', for example, the English surgeon Alexander Francis advocated the 'Francis treatment' or nasal cautery, a procedure that Proust had undergone as a child; according to Francis, cauterizing the nasal mucosa stabilized the 'vasomotor centre'.[52] At the same time, prescription medicines approved by orthodox practitioners did not entirely displace various alternative, and sometimes traditional, popular treatments. During the 1920s and 1930s, a variety of both long-established and novel alternative remedies were endorsed. Noting the tendency for chronic asthmatics to develop a 'barrel-shape' chest as the result of continued over-distension, the Asthma Research Council, for example, advocated remedial physical exercises to 'restore the lungs and chest cavity to their normal size'. Echoing ancient and medieval advice to asthmatics, particularly evident in the writings of Maimonides, the Council's booklet suggested that recurrent or impending attacks of asthma could be prevented by performing 'simple exercises gently'. Similarly, Alexander Gunn Auld advocated swimming 'as an ideal form of exercise for asthmatics', since it deepened breathing, exercised the accessory muscles, and acted as a tonic to the nervous system, and some Indian physicians recommended breathing exercises in conjunction with drugs and desensitization.[53]

Regimen and diet also featured in some early twentieth-century approaches to asthma. In 1936, Harry Benjamin (1885–1986), the German-born sexologist renowned for his work on trans-sexualism, published *Everybody's Guide to Nature Cure*. According to Benjamin, treating asthma 'along orthodox medical lines' not only failed to cure patients, but also threatened to damage their health further with 'highly dangerous' drugs. Instead, Benjamin advocated a natural method of constitutional treatment that aimed to purify 'the system of the toxic matter which is at the root of the trouble': with 'patience and perseverance', he argued, fresh air, gentle outdoor exercise, a carefully monitored diet rich in fruit and vegetables and free from sugars and refined cereals, combined with occasional purgatives, ensured good results.[54]

As the American allergist Francis Rackemann acknowledged in an appendix to his study of clinical allergy published in 1931, a wide range of patent remedies was also available to distressed asthmatics, who, according to Berkart, had been thrown into the 'arms of quacks' by the absence of a rational treatment for the condition: the sickroom at Ferdinand Mount's school, for example, was 'thick with the fumes of Potter's Asthma Cigarettes'.[55] In most cases, commercial nostrums and powders incorporated a variety of familiar ingredients, including stramonium, lobelia, potassium nitrate, potassium iodide, and caffeine. Manufactured and distributed both in America and Europe, 'Felsol', for example, contained phenazone, anilipyrine, jodopyrine, caffeine, and lobelia. According to publicity material, 'Felsol' was not only effective in chronic bronchitis but was also considerably superior to adrenaline in the treatment of asthma. Similarly, chemical analysis of Kellogg's Asthma Powder revealed that it contained stramonium and potassium nitrate. The enduring popularity of these patent remedies, as well as growing interest in the psychological causes of asthma, suggests that, in spite of considerable advances in physiology and pharmacology, many asthmatics were still struggling to breathe.

Asthma and emotions

A close relationship between asthma and the mind had been recognized since antiquity. Indeed, Homer's image of the distraught and asthmatic Hector, panting with exertion on the battlefield, alluded to the emotional, as well as the physical, sources of respiratory distress. During the medieval and early modern periods, writers on asthma such as Maimonides, van Helmont, Floyer, Buchan, and Cullen had routinely stressed both the potential for 'violent passions of the mind' to trigger asthma attacks and the importance of avoiding or subduing excessive anger and fear in patients predisposed to the condition. In the nineteenth century, Salter and others had continued to articulate a traditional belief that both strong emotions and fatigue could initiate or exacerbate asthmatic paroxysms. Historically, the link between emotions and asthma has perhaps constituted one of the least contentious aspects of the disease.

Early twentieth-century reformulations of asthma in terms of allergy failed to undermine the perceived correlation between asthma and the mind. On the contrary, the two theories of asthma were often explored in tandem: initial studies of the psychogenic aspects of asthma were often carried out in allergy clinics and tended to merge psychological and immunological approaches to the disease. In the 1930s, the German physician Erich Wittkower (1899–1983) published the results of his investigations into the 'allergic personality'. Wittkower, who was working at the time at the Tavistock Clinic in London and who later became Professor of Psychiatry at McGill University in Canada and President of the American Psychosomatic Society, compared fifty-five patients from John Freeman's allergy clinic at St Mary's Hospital in London with a similar number of control subjects.[56] Wittkower's conclusion that the typical allergy patient was a delicate, upper-class only child who developed into a socially and emotionally maladjusted adult not only reflected persistent, albeit contested, images of elite, neurotic hay-fever patients, but also legitimated wider cultural stereotypes of the isolated, delicate asthmatic child. In William Golding's *Lord of the Flies*, first published in 1954, the asthmatic Piggy was bespectacled, overweight, and routinely ignored by his fellow castaways.

Parallel clinical studies on both sides of the Atlantic continued to emphasize the emotional determinants of asthma. In Britain during the 1920s, Arthur Hurst and Humphry Rolleston both explored cases of 'hysterical and emotional asthma', in which an 'irritable bronchial centre' was stimulated not only by a familiar array of physical irritants, but by psychological factors such as excitement and worry. Similarly, prominent North American allergists such as Horace S. Baldwin (1895–1983), who based his studies on patients attending the Asthma Department at Cornell University Medical College, New York, suggested that asthma attacks could be triggered by the strain, fatigue, depression, and worry brought on by caring for sick relatives, family arguments, or marital problems. Perhaps more strikingly, the Scottish physician and playwright James Lorimer Halliday (1897–1983) regarded asthma as 'a bodily manifestation of emotional reaction', usually precipitated in the first instance by a perceived threat to life. For Halliday, asthma constituted 'a form of speech, a condensed language of the animal world', an audible symbol of psychological distress that doctors needed to understand and interpret in order to effect a cure.[57]

Increasing clinical interest in the psychological determinants of asthma during the middle decades of the twentieth century was driven partly by the limited impact of new immunological and pharmacological approaches to treatment and partly by the emergence of psychosomatic medicine, especially in North America. Promoted initially by the Hungarian-born analyst Franz Alexander (1891–1964) and the American psychiatrist Helen Flanders Dunbar (1902–59), psychosomatic medicine drew heavily on the theories and approaches of Freudian psychoanalysis as well as on the physiological studies of emotions carried out by Walter Cannon (1871–1945) and others during the inter-war years. Committed to exploring the links between mind and body more carefully, Alexander and Dunbar founded a new journal, *Psychosomatic Medicine*, in 1939 and three years later established a professional organization that eventually became known as the American Psychosomatic Society.

From the start, asthma constituted a central focus for advocates of psychosomatic medicine. According to Alexander and his colleagues, asthma was one of the 'magic seven' psychosomatic conditions, alongside essential hypertension, rheumatoid arthritis, peptic ulceration, ulcerative colitis, hyperthyroidism, and neurodermatitis. Accordingly, early contributions to *Psychosomatic Medicine* attempted to determine the frequency with which emotional factors either precipitated or exacerbated asthma attacks. This approach was not confined to psychiatrists. Although some allergists resisted suggestions that all asthma was psychosomatic, many acknowledged that psychogenic factors contributed to the appearance of the disease. Indeed, according to the English-born allergist Ethan Allan Brown, who became president of the American Academy of Allergy, psychosomatic formulations of asthma promised a more 'satisfactory understanding of its symptomatology' than what he regarded as 'sterile neurological concepts'.[58]

Although proponents of psychosomatic medicine did not entirely dismiss exposure to allergens or inheritance as causative factors, they preferred to prioritize the psychological determinants of asthma and other allergies. For Alexander, the asthmatic wheeze constituted the 'suppressed cry' of a patient suffocated by an over-attentive mother. This image was developed further by Dunbar, particularly in her popular account of psychosomatic medicine, *Mind and Body*, published in 1947. According to Dunbar, the origins of most diseases could be traced to traumatic childhood experiences. Within this context, asthma, hay fever, and eczema were all linked to emotional, and often explicitly sexual, conflicts in childhood:

There are certain specific emotions which seem to be linked
especially to asthma and hay fever. A conflict about longing
for mother love and mother care is one of them. There may
be a feeling of frustration as a result of too little love or a fear
of being smothered by too much. A second emotional conflict characteristic of the allergic is that which results from
suppressed libidinal desire, often closely associated with the
longing for mother. The steady repetition of this emotional
history of 'smother love' in the asthmatic is as marked as the
contrasting history of hostility and unresolved emotional
conflict in the sufferer from hypertension.[59]

Given the deeply buried psychological roots of asthma, only
prolonged and effective psychotherapy, leading to the 'acquisi-
tion of emotional stability', would allow Dunbar's patients to
'breathe again'.[60]

These novel psychoanalytical interpretations of asthma
were not confined to North America. In Britain, both Margaret
Lowenfeld (1890–1973), from the Institute of Child Psychology,
and Theodora Alcock (1888–1980), working at the Tavistock
Clinic of Human Relations in London, studied the personality
characteristics of asthmatic children. Echoing Dunbar's recognition of the interdependence of allergic constitution and
emotional environment, both Lowenfeld and Alcock regarded
asthma as the product of emotional tensions generated particularly by a smothering relationship between patients and their
mothers, a speculation that found support in the life of prominent asthmatics such as Marcel Proust. Significantly, such interpretations were also evident in East Asia. Like their Western
counterparts, many Japanese physicians regarded both nervous
complaints (*kan no mushi*) in young infants and the subsequent
appearance of asthma and other allergies in the same children
as the 'result of overindulgent and overprotective mothering'.[61]

In Europe, alternative visions of mind–body interactions shaped understandings of allergies. According to the Austrian physician Erwin Pulay, for example, hypersensitivity reactions were mediated primarily by the endocrine glands. In *Allergic Man*, first published in German in 1936 and appearing in English in 1945, Pulay suggested that both physical and psychological idiosyncrasies were determined by the balance and function of the sex hormones: allergies, including asthma, were the product of 'a disturbance of equilibrium among the sexual hormones', or what Pulay referred to as an 'intersexual state'. Although Pulay's approach remained marginal, his suggestion that allergy was linked to hormonal balance clearly echoed scientific explorations of allergic mechanisms. Equally, his view that hypersensitivity was associated with intellectual and creative brilliance reinforced enduring presumptions that asthma and hay fever constituted elite diseases of advanced civilization.[62]

Leading European allergists were also interested in the emotional determinants of asthma. Although John Freeman rejected the notion that allergy was 'all nerves' and was critical of overtly Freudian interpretations of allergies, he accepted that 'emotions, moods or tensions are always part of the story'. More particularly, Freeman acknowledged the pivotal role of the emotional, as well as physical, aspects of the domestic environment in provoking or aggravating asthma attacks in susceptible patients. 'Asthmogenic homes' or 'asthmogenic families', he suggested, were those marked by nervous and emotional friction and by excessive parental attention, thereby generating 'emotional infantilism' in the children. Echoing parallel contemporary preoccupations with the role of mothers in shaping tendencies to a variety of conditions, including schizophrenia, anorexia, maladjustment, and delinquency, Freeman concluded that the 'extraordinary prevalence of the Only Child' in his clinics was the result of the emotional suffocation of single children by interfering and 'fussy' mothers, who were bombarded with 'incessant propaganda' about how best to rear their families.[63]

Psychosomatic formulations of asthma were employed to legitimate particular forms of clinical intervention. While some clinicians advocated hypnosis, which was reportedly capable of abrogating hypersensitivity reactions,[64] others suggested the more radical measure of removing asthmatic children from supposedly emotionally disordered homes. Parentectomy (literally, cutting out the parent), as it became known, was pioneered during the 1940s by the American allergist M. Murray Peshkin (1892–1980), who established the Jewish National Home for Asthmatic Children in Denver (later the Children's Asthma Research Institute and Hospital) in order to treat children with intractable asthma. Separation from the home environment offered both reduced exposure to physical allergens and escape from the 'asthmatogenic emotional climate which existed in the child's own home'. According to Peshkin's reports, residence in the institution at Denver led to substantial or complete relief from asthma in 99 per cent of children.[65]

Physicians elsewhere were more cautious about the values of parentectomy than Peshkin and his American colleagues, largely because of anxieties both about oversimplifying the complex and capricious nature of asthma and about removing children indiscriminately from their families and homes. Nevertheless, residential treatments for asthma did become popular in many countries during the middle decades of the twentieth century. In Britain, many asthmatic children were sent to open-air schools in rural or coastal settings or were temporarily relocated to settlements in mountainous areas of Europe, such as Davos in Switzerland or Font Remeu in the Pyrenees. Initially devised during the early twentieth century for children with tuberculosis and bronchitis, both residential institutions and day schools became part of the standard treatment for children with asthma during the middle decades of the twentieth century. Although some American asthmatics later denounced parentectomy as 'one of the most shameful treatments foisted on the sufferers of any disease',[66] life in open-air schools was not universally detested by the children themselves: many of the children sent to schools in the countryside around Birmingham in England during the first half of the twentieth century remember their time with some affection: 'As a child I suffered from bronchial asthma and was sent to Marsh Hill, which I enjoyed very much.'[67]

The benefits of open-air treatment included fresh air, a simple diet, and regular exercise. Similar institutions operated in the southern hemisphere. When the Australian novelist and playwright Patrick White (1912–90) was awarded the Nobel Prize in 1973, he recounted his experiences of asthma as a child and its impact on his creativity:

> My childhood was a sickly one. It was found that I was suffering from nothing worse than asthma, but even so, nobody would insure my life. As a result of the asthma I was sent to school in the country, and only visited Sydney for brief, violently asthmatic sojourns on my way to a house we owned in the Blue Mountains. Probably induced by the asthma, I started reading and writing early on, my literary efforts from the age of about nine running chiefly to poetry and plays.[68]

White's autobiographical reflections also reveal the multifaceted nature of mid-twentieth-century understandings of asthma in terms of both environmental exposure and psychological pressure:

> The hollow in which we lived, or perhaps the pollen from the paspalum which was always threatening to engulf us, or the suspicion that my life had taken a wrong turning, encouraged the worst attacks of asthma I had so far experienced. In the eighteen years we spent at Castle Hill, enslaved more than anything by the trees we had planted, I was in and out of hospitals.[69]

The popularity of psychosomatic approaches to asthma, particularly during the 1940s and 1950s, reflected a particular social and cultural context. On the one hand, psychodynamic interpretations of the impact of mothers and families on health echoed and reinforced reactionary attempts to ensure that women stayed at home to rebuild families and re-establish domestic and social stability in the aftermath of the Second World War: in the wake of the problems caused by evacuation and homelessness amongst children during the conflict, mothers were now needed to restore the mental and physical health of the nation. At the same time, psychosomatic theories were also mobilized in radical holistic critiques of biomedical reductionism. Drawing on growing dissatisfaction with clinical approaches that prioritized somatic over psychological understandings of disease, proponents of psychosocial medicine, such as Halliday, argued that an effective solution to apparently rising levels of psychosomatic diseases required post-war societies not only to combine psychological with physical approaches to disease, but also to expose and challenge the market economy characteristic of Western capitalist societies. As Patrick White's recollections on his life and health make clear, in addition to substantially recasting medical and popular understandings of asthma, these political and professional agendas also profoundly shaped the lives of many young asthmatics.

During the first half of the twentieth century, then, the emergence of novel allergic and psychodynamic theories of asthma tended to overshadow the more specific debates about the relative roles of nervous spasm and mucous obstruction that had preoccupied earlier generations of pathologists, clinicians, and patients. Asthma was increasingly regarded as the product of both inflammation and bronchospasm, which could be triggered either by exposure to allergens or by psychological conflict, or more commonly by a combination of the two. In both cases, clinical preoccupations with the internal physiological and psychological mechanisms involved in asthma served not only to direct attention away from simplistic environmental approaches to the disease and towards more nuanced accounts of individual and familial susceptibility, but also to promote clinical and commercial interest in the development of new pharmacological and analytical approaches to alleviating asthma.

The Second World War constituted a significant turning point in professional and political awareness of the socioeconomic and personal impact of asthma. Anxious about the number of work days lost through illness, during the early 1940s American training schools for nurses listed asthma as one of the conditions that precluded selection for nurse training, along with tuberculosis, obesity, hyperthyroidism, heart disease, and hypertension. Similarly, official investigations into the health of disabled American servicemen carried out in the 1950s revealed not only that several thousand veterans from the First World War had been admitted to army or navy hospitals with asthma and were continuing to receive pensions, but also that asthma constituted

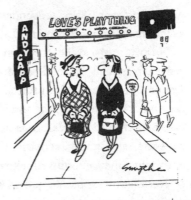

12. A cartoon by Reg Smythe from the *Daily Mirror*, 1958. *(Centre for the Study of Cartoons and Caricature, Templeman Library, University of Kent, copyright Mirrorpix, 1958, reproduced by permission of Mirrorpix)*

"IT WAS 'THRILLIN' THE WAY ANDY USED TO BREATHE 'EAVY WI' EMOTION — LATER ON I FOUND IT WAS ASTHMA"

one of the principal grounds for medical discharge from the services during the Second World War and a continuing cause of respiratory ill health. In order to improve the clinical facilities available for asthmatic servicemen, the American Academy of Allergy encouraged the secondment of allergists to service hospitals, developed training courses for military medical officers, and subsequently established a Military Allergists Committee.[70]

In the decades following the Second World War, poets and cartoonists continued to exploit the symbolic and metaphorical richness of psychosomatic accounts of asthma: in the confessional poetry of Anne Sexton (1928–74), the laboured breathing of asthmatics signified the emotional desolation of suburban marriage; and in Reg Smythe's Andy Capp cartoon published in the *Daily Mirror* in 1958, asthma was satirized as the embodiment of passion and love.[71] However, in many ways recognition of the military significance of asthma, together with the availability of more potent anti-asthma medication, contributed to the declining popularity of psychosomatic formulations of asthma in the post-war period. Although some writers continued to recommend rural retreats or 'health villages' for the treatment of both the physical and the emotional elements of asthma, and although asthma retained its status as the archetypal psychosomatic disorder well into the 1980s, in general psychological strategies were eclipsed by biological and pharmacological approaches to the disease. Indeed, in several countries the parents of asthmatic children, as well as the patients themselves, began to challenge assumptions that mothers and families were to blame or that parentectomy offered a humane solution to childhood asthma. Members of the Asthma Foundation of New South Wales in Australia and supporters of Nancy Sander's pioneering Mothers of Asthmatics set up in North America in 1985, for example, campaigned to dispel what they regarded as a variety of harmful, stigmatizing myths about the psychological and domestic determinants of asthma and to promote more balanced scientific understandings of the condition.[72]

In contrast to the fate of psychosomatic approaches, the notion of allergy gained considerable currency, providing the conceptual tools for innovative therapeutic interventions aimed at manipulating what were regarded as aberrant, idiosyncratic responses to external allergens. From the first decade of the twentieth century, rising trends in allergic diseases and the growth of clinical allergy had provided American and European pharmaceutical companies with both the motive and the opportunity to develop profitable new treatments for asthma, hay fever, and eczema, such as desensitizing vaccines, ephedrine, aminophylline, adrenaline, and corticosteroids. During the decades following the Second World War, clarification of the mechanisms and mediators of allergic reactions, including the discovery of IgE, the antibody responsible for initiating many clinical manifestations of hypersensitivity, provided further impetus for an expanding multinational pharmaceutical industry to invest substantial resources in developing and marketing anti-asthma and anti-allergy drugs. Paradoxically, it was arguably this drive to identify and implement pharmaceutical solutions to the persistent personal problems experienced by asthmatics that unleashed a tragedy that transformed the character and meaning of asthma in the second half of the twentieth century.

IV

ASTHMA IN THE MODERN WORLD

On a bad day I feel like I'm drowning and I can't reach the surface of the water and I am going to burst, yet a tiny, tiny bit of air keeps me alive. It's very scary—I feel like I'm living with a time bomb and if I have a bad attack I say to myself: 'Is this the one that will kill me?'

Catherine Tunnicliffe, in Asthma UK, *Living on a Knife Edge*, 2004

On Saturday, 7 June 2008, at the onset of the monsoon period marked by the Hindu ritual of Mrigasari Karti, several thousand people with asthma arrived in Hyderabad in India in order to receive a controversial treatment for their respiratory illness. For over 160 years, the Bathini Goud family had been dispensing a secret remedy that had reportedly been revealed to one of their ancestors by a saint in 1845 on the condition that the medicine would be administered without cost to all patients. The treatment, which comprised swallowing a live murrel fish stuffed with a yellow medicinal paste, was referred to by the Goud family as a 'fish prasadam', a form of karma-free food offered to the gods. According to popular belief, consumption of the medicine, followed by a strict diet for forty-five days, for three successive years effectively prevents the accumulation of phlegm and offers a complete cure for asthma.

The fish treatment for asthma has been the subject of considerable dispute in recent years. In addition to the crowds of asthmatics who travel long distances and patiently queue for a cure every June, the treatment has been endorsed by prominent members of the Bharatiya Janata Party, a right-wing Hindu political organization that has persistently supported practitioners of traditional āyurvedic medicine. After chemical analysis revealed that the herbal paste contained familiar āyurvedic anti-asthma remedies such as asafoetida, turmeric, and jaggery, the state-funded Department of Ayurveda, Yoga and Naturopathy, Unani, Siddha and Homoeopathy (AYUSH) also tentatively concluded that the medicine was potentially useful to asthma patients.

Conversely, a number of physicians have not only criticized the Goud family for failing to reveal the ingredients of the medicine as required by the terms of the Drugs and Magical Remedies Act 1954, but have also insisted that the treatment is ineffective. According to Dr Ajit Vigg, director of respiratory and critical care medicine at a hospital in Hyderabad, in 'my practice of 20–25 years, I have not seen a single patient whose condition has either improved or who has got completely cured with fish medicine'.[1] In 2004, growing professional and political concerns about the safety and efficacy of the Goud's secret asthma remedy prompted the Indian Medical Association to challenge the treatment in court. The resulting laboratory tests, ordered by the Hyderabad High Court, not only revealed the presence of active āyurvedic ingredients in the herbal paste, but also rejected critics' claims that the preparation contained steroids or harmful substances. The outcome of the investigation was a compromise: regarded as a therapy but not a medicine, the fish treatment continues to be dispensed although without official state support.

The recent history of the fish remedy is instructive. At one level, the popularity of the treatment in India testifies to the shifting epidemiology of asthma in the modern world. Once regarded as the preserve of advanced industrial civilizations, asthma now figures prominently in the morbidity and mortality statistics from developing countries: there are an estimated 15–20 million people with asthma in India alone. Equally, asthma no longer afflicts only the affluent elite as many late-nineteenth- and early twentieth-century medical authorities had assumed; on the contrary, like many chronic diseases, asthma is now more common and more commonly fatal amongst impoverished and deprived social groups.

At another level, virulent disputes about the fish remedy reveal a close relationship between the rising prevalence and severity of asthma, on the one hand, and broader political, professional, and economic interests, on the other. In addition to betraying a lack of faith in the powers of modern Western medicine to alleviate or cure asthma, persistent public demand for the fish treatment, along with many other less conventional remedies such as acupuncture, hypnosis, homoeopathy, restricted diets, and breathing exercises, exemplifies the contested boundaries between supposedly orthodox and alternative systems of medicine. Economic factors occupy the heart of such disputes: at the start of the twenty-first century, asthma carries both the prospect of substantial profit and the spectre of financial loss for multinational pharmaceutical companies, employers, national health services, the cleaning industry, and food retailers.

Such tensions between the interests of patients, practitioners, and industry are evident in more personal accounts of asthma. In the 1990s, driven by a desire to understand and control his own illness, the radio commentator Tim Brookes published his reflections on the manifestations, meanings, and management of asthma. Starting with a vivid description of a severe asthma attack that echoed the intimate revelations of many earlier asthmatics such as John Floyer and Marcel Proust, Brookes's narrative makes clear the terrifying impact of the disease in both acute and chronic forms:

> Everything was closing in around my throat and chest; I felt a frightening internal claustrophobia, a sense of metabolic urgency rapidly mounting toward panic...Over the years, I came to recognize several kinds of asthma: most were a lighter or heavier wheeze that came on gradually late in the evening, or more suddenly when shoveling snow in a heavy coat. These attacks sounded like the word *asthma*, a sibilant rasp. Three times since I'd turned thirty, though, something entirely different had happened, a sudden, overwhelming assault that stormed through my whole body, seizing my throat and suffocating me. This felt like one of those asthmas.[2]

According to Brookes, Western scientific medicine offered only limited assistance in his quest to explain and cure his illness: 'But the more questions I asked, the fewer answers came back. Asthma seemed to have the medical community in turmoil.' Having explored a wide range of explanations and treatments for his condition, Brookes ultimately recommended pursuing an alternative clinical path that not only exploits modern scientific knowledge but also acknowledges the links between illness and identity that were often recognized by doctors from an earlier age: 'Medicine needs a pre-specialist goal, a new, unifying sense of purpose to match the emerging understanding of our subtle and complex relationship with illness. Medicine, I think, needs to be seen as a meeting between patient and physician, on equal footing, in the real world, with the aim of promoting self-understanding.'[3]

This final chapter explores the epidemiological and personal features of asthma in the modern world. By examining in turn changing patterns of mortality, rising global trends in morbidity, and the intimate relationship between asthma and industry, this chapter addresses two striking paradoxes in the recent history of the disease. First, it is evident that the prevalence and severity of asthma rose substantially during the last half of the twentieth century in spite of developments in pharmaceutical treatment and clinical management: as medical science advanced, chronic illness and death appeared to flourish. Secondly, it is noticeable that, as scientific knowledge of the aetiology and pathogenesis of asthma deepened, the definition of the condition became less stable. Although attempts to identify asthma in terms of reversible bronchial hyper-reactivity and intermittent airway obstruction have helped to integrate disparate clinical accounts of the disease, several types of asthma have continued to coexist. Not only do different people experience and manifest asthma in contrasting ways, but asthma is also measured and determined by a wide range of conflicting diagnostic tests: asthma can be revealed by subjective accounts of respiratory symptoms such as wheeze, nocturnal cough, and breathlessness, by raised levels of IgE, allergy skin prick tests, and eosinophilia, by the demonstration of reduced lung function such as diminished forced expiratory volume (FEV) and peak expiratory flow (PEF), and by the response to treatment with bronchodilators. At the dawn of the new millennium, multiple and contested versions of asthma persist much as they did in earlier times.

Deaths from asthma

Prior to the Second World War, many clinicians possessed a relatively benign image of asthma. According to Archie Norman, who trained in medicine during the inter-war years and who subsequently established a Respiratory Unit at Great Ormond Street Hospital, London, in the 1950s, 'asthma in childhood then was very much what you might call an "orphan disease". Nobody was that interested in it. There was no adequate treatment and children didn't ordinarily die from it, so the principal physicians really tended to pay it little attention.'[4] As John Morrison Smith (1918–2001), a consultant chest physician in Birmingham, acknowledged in his retrospective reflections on the treatment of asthma, one consequence of this lack of clinical attention during the 1930s and 1940s was that doctors subsequently found themselves ill-equipped to deal with patients:

> It is difficult to appreciate today the feeling of helplessness
> I remember just over 30 years ago when, having recently
> obtained a senior appointment, I was consulted by an intelli-
> gent young man with severe asthma. He had failed to respond
> to bronchodilators and his distress was such as to threaten
> his otherwise happy and successful family and business life.
> It was apparent to me, and to him, that my scanty teaching
> on the subject as an undergraduate and even 11 years' experi-
> ence in practice had not prepared me for this problem.[5]

Reinforced by prominent cultural representations of asthma and hay fever as mild diseases of the privileged classes, professional disinterest persisted into the post-war years. According to a medical guide for captains of ships, published in 1952 by the British Ministry of Transport, asthma was 'often very distressing', but not 'a dangerous disease'.[6] In the early 1960s, however, reassuring clinical perceptions of asthma were undermined by epidemiological evidence indicating that the prevalence and severity of asthma were beginning to rise. Although international statistics suggested that deaths from asthma had declined during the 1950s, a number of factors served to reverse that trend and alert both patients and their doctors to the potential fatality of the disease. A wave of deaths from asthma amongst young adults in Britain, rising trends in morbidity and mortality from asthma amongst socially deprived ethnic minorities in several North American cities, and a surge of asthma and deaths from asthma following an industrial air pollution episode in Japan in 1961 collectively served to reorient professional and public attitudes.

In an article in the *British Medical Journal* published in 1997, a Scottish general practitioner, James McCracken (1930–2005), reflected on a fatal case of asthma that he had witnessed while working as a locum in the Scottish Highlands in the late 1950s. Called to attend a 16-year-old girl who was suffering from an asthma attack in the middle of the night, McCracken arrived at the house confident that he 'knew all about asthma' and that he would be able to manage the situation, if necessary by administering a subcutaneous injection of adrenaline. To his dismay, he discovered that the girl was already dead: 'I went home a chastened man. I found that I knew less about asthma than I thought I knew.'[7]

Over the next few years, this tragic outcome was to be reproduced in homes and hospitals throughout Britain. In an article published in the *Lancet* in 1966, John Morrison Smith warned that asthma deaths had increased by more than 50 per cent during the first five years of the decade, with the most marked rise occurring in children over 5 years old. More detailed epidemiological analysis soon revealed an epidemic of asthma deaths, particularly in England and Wales. From 1959, asthma mortality had risen steadily in all age groups, although the trend was especially evident in children between 10 and 14 years old, at which ages the mortality rate had increased eightfold between 1959 and 1966. In addition, studies revealed that the proportion of all deaths between the ages of 5 and 34 that were attributable to asthma had risen from 1 per cent in 1959 to 3.4 per cent in 1966; in children between 10 and 14 years old, the proportional mortality had increased even more dramatically, from 1 per cent in 1959 to 7.2 per cent in 1966. By 1966, asthma had become the fourth most common cause of death, exceeded in children only by road-traffic accidents, cancer, and respiratory infections.[8]

According to W. H. W. Inman (1929–2005), Senior Medical Officer to the Committee on Safety of Drugs and one of the principal commentators on asthma mortality in Britain at that time, the wave of asthma deaths initially constituted a 'silent epidemic' that attracted only minimal professional and press attention.[9] However, by the late 1960s a number of articles had appeared in *The Times* not only pointing to the tragic irony that better management of asthma since the war had not resulted in a fall in mortality, but also alerting readers to the alarm that the epidemic was causing amongst patients and doctors. In addition, newspaper coverage noted that rising mortality from asthma was not confined to England and Wales, but was also evident in certain other industrialized countries; similar waves of asthma deaths were reported in Australia, New Zealand,

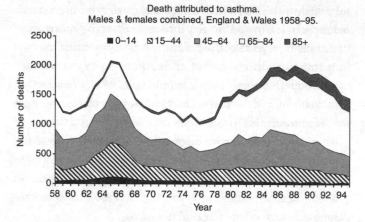

Death attributed to asthma.
Males & females combined, England & Wales 1958–95.

13. Asthma mortality rates in England and Wales. (*Crown copyright, reproduced from the Lung and Asthma Information Agency Factsheets 97/3 and 2001/1, http://www.sghms.ac.uk/depts/laia/laia.htm*)

Scotland, Ireland, and Norway. Towards the end of the decade, growing public and professional concerns encouraged epidemiologists to analyse the patterns of mortality more closely across space and time in order to identify a possible cause for rising deaths from asthma.

There were a number of possible explanations for post-war trends in mortality. In the first place, it was possible that the sudden rise in asthma fatalities merely constituted an artefact created by changes in diagnostic practice. From the late 1950s, pathologists and physicians had certainly attempted to establish a clearer definition of asthma and to distinguish more accurately between asthma, chronic bronchitis, and emphysema. Drawing partly on the availability of new treatments and partly on developments in the measurement of lung function, such as the introduction of the peak flow meter by Martin Wright in

1959, many researchers increasingly regarded asthma primarily in functional terms as a form of intermittent airway obstruction that could be reversed by bronchodilators. By contrast, chronic bronchitis was defined largely in clinical terms by the presence of a productive cough, while emphysema was characterized principally on a pathological basis as dilatation of the air-spaces distal to the terminal bronchioles.[10]

There is some evidence to suggest that shifting understandings of chronic respiratory diseases in these terms did indeed lead to changes in diagnostic practice in some countries, and especially to the adoption of asthma as a label to describe cases previously diagnosed as bronchitis. In a survey of allergic diseases in general practice published in 1972, for example, J. M. Perkin observed that 'many of the patients ultimately diagnosed as extrinsic asthma had in fact been labelled as recurrent wheezy bronchitis initially'.[11] Similarly, while reviewing his own experiences as a general practitioner during the 1960s and 1970s, Denis Pereira Gray, later president of the Royal College of General Practitioners, noted in 1979 that 'I find now that what I used to call bronchitis is usually asthma'.[12] Yet, according to early epidemiological studies, shifting diagnostic practices could not satisfactorily explain mortality trends in the 1960s; since deaths attributable to other chronic respiratory diseases did not decrease while asthma deaths were rising, the increase in asthma mortality could not be construed simply in terms of classificatory changes. On the contrary, the evidence suggested that the wave of asthma mortality was 'in large part, real and represents a true increase in the annual number of deaths from the disease'.[13]

Early studies also rejected the possibility that rising mortality could be explained simply in terms of an increase in the number of patients suffering from asthma or in terms of alterations in the levels of environmental pollutants. Instead, they tentatively suggested that advances in the management of respiratory diseases might be responsible. In particular, researchers began to notice a close correlation between mortality rates and 'the use of pressurized aerosols containing sympathomimetics', such as the β-agonists isoprenaline or orciprenaline, used to relieve the characteristic bronchospasm of an asthma attack. High-dose forms of these relatively non-selective bronchodilators had become more widely available and more commonly used during the late 1950s and early 1960s following the introduction of the first metered dose inhaler, developed by Riker Laboratories in 1956; by 1966, consumption of non-selective bronchodilators had increased more than fourfold.[14] As epidemiological studies subsequently demonstrated, not only did the onset of the epidemic coincide with the introduction of this form of treatment, but mortality rates also rapidly subsided once the use of these preparations declined following warnings from the Committee on Safety of Drugs in 1967 and the eventual proscription of direct sales to the British public under Schedule 4B of the Poisons Regulations in 1968.

Although further enquiries tended to confirm beliefs that the overuse of non-selective β-agonists was largely responsible for the British epidemic of asthma deaths, either because of their directly toxic effect on the heart or because they masked the severity of the attack and led to delays in treatment, the correlation between bronchodilator use and death remained contentious. However, early suspicions of the iatrogenic nature of the British epidemic found indirect support from mortality patterns elsewhere in the world. In 1972, Paul Stolley, from the School of Hygiene and Public Health at the Johns Hopkins University, suggested that many countries, including the United

States, were spared an epidemic largely because they did not market or sell large volumes of the highly concentrated form of isoprenaline that was available in England. In addition, as Neil Pearce has argued, during the late 1970s New Zealand experienced a second wave of asthma deaths apparently linked to the prescription of a high-dose preparation of fenoterol, another relatively non-selective β-agonist. In a manner analogous to the mortality pattern in the 1960s, this second epidemic began to wane only in 1990 following the withdrawal of fenoterol from the drug tariff.[15]

The British wave of deaths from asthma in the 1960s carried both immediate and long-term consequences. In addition to precipitating tighter regulation of the sale of non-selective bronchodilators such as isoprenaline, the tragedy also discouraged the use of adrenaline and ephedrine, which had constituted the mainstay of treatment for asthma during the inter-war years. At the same time, researchers in the pharmaceutical industry strove to develop more selective bronchodilators, or β_2-agonists, which acted predominantly on smooth muscle in the lungs; as will become apparent, the results of these initiatives effectively ushered in a new era in the treatment of asthma. Deaths from asthma also encouraged both patients and doctors to recognize the potential seriousness of the condition, leading to efforts to improve medical training, introduce guidelines for managing asthma attacks, facilitate self-referral to hospital, establish asthma clinics in general practice, and monitor asthma morbidity and mortality more closely.

While the British epidemic certainly declined in the late 1960s, deaths from asthma did not entirely disappear. As national mortality statistics make clear, approximately 1,500 patients continued to die from asthma each year in England and

Wales throughout the 1970s and 1980s. Subsequent international comparisons suggested that severe, and sometime fatal, asthma continued to plague the British population more than its European counterparts. At the turn of the millennium, mortality from asthma was higher in the United Kingdom than elsewhere in Europe, more common in adults than children, and more frequent in men than women. As these patterns indicate, in certain parts of the modern world asthma possessed a new, life-threatening personality.

Awareness of the increasing severity and impact of asthma was also fostered by experiences elsewhere in the world. Although the United States was spared an epidemic of iatrogenic deaths during the 1960s, certain American cities experienced a dramatic surge in asthma morbidity and mortality during that decade. In 1963, a wave of asthma swept through the Caribbean island of Cuba. Supposedly linked to sudden atmospheric changes, the crisis resulted in the death of five people and the hospitalization of more than 200 others. Two years later, newspapers reported 'a startling rise in asthma...among New York Negroes and Puerto Ricans'. Drawing on contemporary beliefs in the psychosomatic nature of asthma and assumptions about inherent racial predispositions to disease, such outbreaks were initially attributed to 'tensions arising from conditions related directly or indirectly to the civil rights movement'.[16] However, as Gregg Mitman has argued in his provocative analysis of American allergies, interpretations that emphasized the vulnerability of the 'damaged black psyche' were challenged by epidemiological evidence: the prevalence of severe asthma in certain districts of New York, Chicago, and New Orleans was closely correlated with urban poverty and environmental inequalities, and particularly with high levels of cockroach infestation in sub-standard housing.[17] In contrast to earlier images of asthma as a fashionable, elite disease of civilization, modern American asthma was a manifestation of social deprivation.

By the 1970s, the outbreak of American asthma had declined as widespread race riots eventually triggered improvements in the quality of housing stock and medical care in urban ghettos. However, a link between asthma and race persisted. Recent studies have suggested that approximately 20 per cent of the population in Barbados suffers from asthma. As Ian Whitmarsh has argued, this figure cannot be explained simply in terms of biology and race, as some commentators have suggested; both asthma and race are ambiguous and contested entities that need to be understood within a particular socioeconomic context. High levels of recorded asthma amongst Afro-Caribbeans in Barbados thus reflect genetic differences, local diagnostic practices, industrial pharmaceutical pressures, government policies, and cultural expectations.[18] In this sense, the term 'asthma' continues to encapsulate, and articulate between, a diverse range of personal experiences, professional interests, and political agendas.

As the American and Caribbean cases suggest, post-war trends in asthma morbidity and mortality appeared to be closely associated with social and economic conditions. Further support for this came from Japan during the early 1960s. Following the ravages of the Second World War, the Japanese government initiated a widespread programme of social and economic recovery. Rapid industrialization and urbanization, combined with the introduction of mass-production techniques, served to reconfigure the Japanese landscape. Although effective in economic terms, the growth of Japanese industry during this period carried severe environmental consequences: during the

1950s and 1960s, the air became heavily polluted with industrial dusts and acid gases, and the coastlines, waterways and countryside despoiled by waste. In the process, the health of both humans and animals was severely compromised.

Pollution-related diseases had appeared in Japan during the inter-war years: Minamata disease was linked to poisoning with mercury released from the Chisso chemical factory; and Itai-Itai disease occurred in the mining district of the Toyama Prefecture as the result of cadmium poisoning. In addition, in the 1940s, North American military doctors had described a form of 'asthmatic bronchitis', or 'Tokyo–Yokohama asthma', marked by wheezing, coughing, and dyspnoea, that had affected air-force personnel and their families stationed on the heavily polluted Kanto Plain region south of Tokyo.[19] However, the public health impact of industrialization deepened in the 1950s and 1960s following the rapid growth of the Japanese petrochemical industry. As the Showa Yokkaichi Oil company expanded, greater levels of sulphurous gases were released into the atmosphere, leading to a dramatic rise in asthma and respiratory distress. The first cases of 'Yokkaichi asthma' were described in 1961 and over subsequent years resulted in several deaths and considerable morbidity. Although increased public and political agitation, including lawsuits against the petrochemical companies, served to initiate new environmental protection programmes in Japan during the 1970s, there is some evidence that many patients continue to suffer increased mortality and decreased life-expectancy as a late effect of exposure to air pollution in the 1960s.[20]

It is not clear precisely how to evaluate the wave of severe asthma that killed patients and traumatized families and communities throughout the world during the 1960s. It is possible that rising deaths from asthma signalled a new, more malignant form of the disease, one effectively generated by pharmaceutical innovation, industrial pollution, and social injustice. It is also possible that the post-war epidemic of asthma mortality simply reacquainted modern commentators with an enduring historical truth, recognized by medical writers since antiquity: asthma can kill. However the epidemics are explained, they constituted a critical moment in the transformation of twentieth-century understandings and experiences of the condition. It was no longer realistic for doctors to portray asthma as a mild inconvenience suffered only by the socially and educationally elite. From the 1960s, patients, doctors, and governments were forced to acknowledge that asthma constituted a significant threat to both health and life, particularly amongst socially deprived sections of modern populations.

Global trends in asthma

In addition to raising awareness of the socioeconomic determinants and personal impact of asthma, the epidemics of deaths during the 1960s highlighted long-standing uncertainties about the precise definition and diagnostic indicators of asthma and about its relationship to other respiratory diseases. Since antiquity, asthma had been diagnosed by the association of a particular constellation of symptoms, namely a wheeze and cough accompanied by respiratory distress. However, these symptoms were not specific to asthma and, over the centuries, medical writers had regularly disagreed about the interpretation of conflicting diagnostic tests and about the relative importance of different clinical presentations, such as the contrasting humoral and spasmodic forms of asthma disputed by eighteenth- and nineteenth-century physicians. These dilemmas persisted. In 1971, a group of leading clinicians charged with the task of defining asthma more clearly concluded that the condition could 'not be defined on the information at present available'.[21] More recently, Anne Tattersfield, director of the Division of Respiratory Medicine at the University of Nottingham, and her colleagues have reiterated the difficulties associated with defining and classifying asthma:

> Asthma has no standard definition. Attempts to define asthma have generally resulted in descriptive statements invoking notions of variable airflow obstruction over short periods of time, sometimes in association with markers of airway hyper-responsiveness and cellular pathology of the airway; they have not, however, provided validated quantitative criteria for these characteristics to enable diagnosis of asthma to be standardised for clinical, epidemiological, or genetic purposes.[22]

As other modern commentators made clear, problems of classification and comparison were related to the complexity of the disease. According to Australian researchers, the 'difficulty in measuring asthma across populations is that the disease is a complex entity with pathologists, physiologists, clinicians, patients, and epidemiologists all having different perspectives'.[23] In order to obviate these difficulties, studies of asthma carried out during the last decades of the twentieth century tended to identify a single measure, such as self-reported levels of wheeze, as a more effective and consistent indicator of asthma prevalence and incidence.

Although differences in diagnosis have made comparisons difficult across time and between countries, epidemiological evidence suggests that asthma became more common

throughout the world during the last half of the twentieth century. Following the initial decline of deaths in the late 1960s,
there was a steady rise in both morbidity and mortality rates
from asthma in England and Wales. In 1995, a survey conducted
by the Department of Health revealed that between the 1970s
and the 1990s there were significant increases in the levels of
self-reported and general-practitioner-reported asthma, in hospital admissions for asthma, and in the number of days of certified incapacity as the result of asthma. According to figures
obtained from national morbidity surveys, the proportion of
the population consulting family doctors for asthma increased
from 8.5 per 1,000 in 1955–6 to 10.2 in 1970–1, and to 17.8 in
1981–2. This trend was supported by a survey conducted in the
west of Scotland, according to which the prevalence of asthma
rose from 3 per cent in 1972 to 8.2 per cent in 1996.[24] By the turn
of the millennium, an estimated 5.2 million people in Britain
suffered from asthma.

The British experience was shared by most developed countries. In the United States, the prevalence of asthma nearly doubled between 1980 and 1994 and hospital admission rates tripled
between 1970 and 1995. At the start of the twenty-first century,
approximately fifteen million Americans suffered from asthma.
In addition to emphasizing the human cost of rising trends in
asthma, North American figures also revealed the deepening economic impact of the disease. In 1985, the total cost of
asthma was already $4.5 billion for in-patient, emergency, and
out-patient care, medical services, medication, loss of work,
and death; by 1992, the cost had risen to $6 billion. Similar
trends in asthma morbidity were evident in Europe, especially
in Scandinavian countries, and in Australasia. In Norway, for
example, asthma rates doubled between 1981 and 1993, while in

Australia, which has one of the highest prevalence rates in the world, the percentage of children aged between 8 and 11 diagnosed with asthma rose from 12.9 per cent in 1982 to 29.7 per cent in 1992.[25]

Towards the end of the twentieth century, attempts to capture changing prevalence rates more accurately were promoted by global collaborative initiatives, such as the International Study of Asthma and Allergies in Childhood (ISAAC) established in 1991 and the Global Initiative for Asthma (GINA) founded in 1993. Before that, most of the international comparative figures had been compiled solely by the World Health Organization (WHO), which had started to investigate the prevalence and socioeconomic impact of allergies during the 1970s and 1980s. The results of WHO surveys were striking. In addition to demonstrating rising trends in asthma in developed countries, studies funded by the WHO also suggested that asthma rates increased in developing countries during the late twentieth century: in Japan, asthma rates doubled between 1955 and 1971; although asthma was relatively uncommon in Africa during the post-war years, it rapidly emerged as a clinical problem in many African countries during the 1970s; and in Papua New Guinea, asthma was extremely rare in the 1960s, but affected 7.3 per cent of the adult population by the 1980s. In some remote locations, such as Tristan da Cunha and the Maldive Islands, asthma prevalence rates were found to exceed those of many Western countries, suggesting that the links between civilization and asthma were more complex than had previously been assumed.[26]

As many researchers warned, however, direct comparisons across space and time remained problematic, with wide variations in prevalence being reported not only between, but also within, countries. In addition, as historical accounts of asthma

in India indicate, interpretation of the statistics requires intimate knowledge of the precise context in which the diagnosis
was being made. According to surveys carried out in Delhi
and Patna in the 1960s, the prevalence of asthma in India was
approximately 2 per cent. By the early 1990s, the rate had
risen to between 3.5 per cent and 6 per cent; in the late 1990s,
studies revealed a further rise in prevalence to approximately
15 per cent. Although these figures appear to reinforce the general argument that asthma prevalence has risen worldwide, they
conceal a more elaborate story.

It is clear that post-Second World War estimates of asthma
prevalence in India were compromised by a number of factors.
In the first instance, the stigma associated with the condition,
which was frequently thought to be contagious, debilitating,
and incurable, led to reluctance on the part of both parents and
physicians to label children asthmatic. As David van Sickle has
argued in his anthropological studies of asthma and allergy in
south India, many doctors preferred to employ terms such as
'wheezy bronchitis' or 'allergic bronchitis' in order to encourage
compliance with treatment, and referred to their out-patient
clinics as 'wheezy child', rather than asthma, clinics.[27] Secondly,
given the heavy burden of tuberculosis and bronchitis in India,
patients presenting with respiratory symptoms were more
frequently diagnosed as suffering from respiratory infections
rather than asthma. In both ways, as some Indian physicians
pointed out, the prevalence of asthma was under-reported during the 1960s and 1970s, a phenomenon that arguably served to
exaggerate the apparent rise of asthma during the later decades
of the twentieth century.[28]

While there was a general consensus that asthma morbidity
and mortality had risen worldwide during the second half of the

twentieth century, there were considerable disputes about the causes of those trends. For many centuries, both doctors and asthmatics had recognized familial tendencies towards asthma. During the early twentieth century, this was interpreted largely in terms of atopy, or an inherited predisposition to allergies. In the decades following the Second World War, evidence of varying prevalence rates between racial groups sharing a common environment, as well as studies of twins and inbred populations, encouraged scientists to search more energetically for the gene or genes that might be responsible for asthma. Several genetic configurations were identified as potential candidates, including polymorphism in the genes coding for the high-affinity receptor for IgE, those coding for the β_2-adrenergic receptor, which was thought to dictate both the severity of asthma and responses to bronchodilator treatment, or those responsible for determining bronchial hyper-reactivity.[29] However, while genetic factors continued to attract both clinical and media attention, most studies suggested that the pace of the global rise in asthma was more likely to be the product of environmental and lifestyle, rather than racial or genetic, factors.

A wide range of environmental factors, linked predominantly to the processes of modernization or 'Westernization', have been implicated in recent trends in asthma. One of the most popular and enduring theories highlights the possible role of air pollution. Urban smoke had been identified as a major health hazard in Britain and other modernizing countries during the Industrial Revolution of the late eighteenth and early nineteenth centuries. As industrial expansion and urbanization led to the increased combustion of coal in domestic as well as manufacturing settings, smoke pollution became a problem not only in large British industrial centres, such as London and Manchester, but also in Europe, North America, Japan, and Australia. From the mid-nineteenth century, the Registrar General regularly attributed excess deaths in London from bronchitis, pneumonia, asthma, and whooping cough to a combination of fog and pollution. These concerns persisted into the early decades of the twentieth century, stimulating the growth of open-air colonies and schools for children with tuberculosis, bronchitis, and asthma, and fuelling the fashion amongst wealthy asthmatics, such as Marcel Proust, for taking holidays in mountainous, coastal, or lakeside 'respiratory resorts', where the air was supposedly cleaner and more invigorating than the polluted urban atmosphere.

Continuing anxieties about the impact of air pollution on health encouraged official state inquiries, facilitated the passage of smoke abatement legislation, and led to the formation of pressure groups campaigning for clean air. Initially, these efforts brought little success. Political reluctance to interfere with industrial interests, persistent beliefs that the urban atmosphere might be of benefit to asthmatics, and continuing ideological commitments to the domestic hearth as a symbol of individual and national prosperity collectively served to undermine arguments for reform. During the middle decades of the twentieth century, however, a number of highly visible international air-pollution episodes, in which large numbers of people died, precipitated government intervention on both sides of the Atlantic. Events in the Meuse Valley in Belgium in 1930, in Donora, Pennsylvania, in 1948, and, perhaps most significantly, in London in 1952 alerted politicians and physicians around the world to the impact of pollution on respiratory and cardiovascular health. In Britain, the Committee on Air Pollution, appointed in the wake of the London smog and chaired by the South African engineer and industrialist Sir Hugh Beaver (1890–1967), reported that, at the height of the smog, deaths from bronchitis had increased ninefold, deaths from pneumonia fourfold, and deaths from other respiratory diseases in the region of five to sixfold. The Committee's report concluded that there was 'a clear association between pollution [especially by smoke and sulphur dioxide] and the incidence of bronchitis and other respiratory diseases'.[30]

Air pollution episodes during the 1940s and 1950s eventually acted as a catalyst for the introduction of clean air policies in both Europe and North America. However, although official inquiries acknowledged the influence of air pollution on bronchitis, pneumonia, and lung cancer, the evidence regarding asthma was equivocal. Neither a report from the Ministry of Health in 1954 nor one published in 1970 by the Royal College of Physicians identified a causative link between urban air pollution, on the one hand, and asthma morbidity and mortality, on the other. Similarly, in spite of evidence suggesting that asthmatics might be more sensitive to lower levels of sulphur dioxide than the rest of the population and that exposure to air pollution, including cigarette smoke, could initiate or exacerbate acute asthma attacks, studies failed to identify a clear link between changing sulphur dioxide concentrations in the atmosphere and the prevalence of asthma.[31]

Doubts about the role of air pollution in asthma were partly driven by observations that, during the period when asthma was increasing, visible atmospheric pollution was declining in most developed countries. In Britain, for example, emissions of sulphur dioxide and black smoke clearly fell in the wake of the Clean Air Acts of 1956 and 1968. As subsequent international studies suggested, however, measures of the effects of pollution on health needed to consider the impact of invisible pollutants from traffic rather than merely industrial processes. From the middle decades of the twentieth century, increased emissions from cars and buses encouraged researchers to evaluate the role of pollutants discharged during petrol and diesel combustion either as initiators of asthma or as factors that could provoke asthma attacks in certain patients. The evidence proved ambiguous. In spite of reports suggesting that vehicle pollution might exacerbate the symptoms of asthma, and in spite of evidence demonstrating the role of pollutants on lung function in animals, links between levels of traffic and trends in asthma have remained speculative and contested. Comparative studies charting the prevalence of asthma in Germany following the removal of the Berlin Wall in 1989 and subsequent political reunification in 1990 showed paradoxically that asthma and other allergies were less common in heavily polluted East German cities than in their West German counterparts.[32] Likewise, several cities or regions with high levels of atmospheric pollution, such as Athens in Greece and parts of China, generally experienced low levels of asthma, while countries with relatively clean air, such as Scotland and New Zealand, demonstrated high rates of asthma during the last half of the twentieth century.

Although the media and various pressure groups continued to expose the ways in which industrial pollution and dirty cities were supposedly fuelling modern Western trends in asthma, scientific reservations about the role of air pollution in shaping modern global patterns of the disease were reinforced by inquiries conducted by national and international committees and by professional organizations. In 1995, a working party of the British Society for Allergy and Clinical Immunology concluded: 'There is limited evidence at the moment to support the

idea that air pollutants are responsible for the increased prevalence of asthma and allergic disease in countries with a "western" lifestyle. Worldwide, where increased incidence of allergic
disease has been convincingly documented over time, allergen
exposure has more obviously been responsible than exposure
to air pollutants.'[33]

It is possible that atmospheric pollution has exerted an indirect effect on the prevalence of asthma through its impact on
climate change and pollen levels. Two Australian researchers, Paul Beggs and Hilary Bambrick, recently suggested that
anthropogenic climate change, most notably raised concentrations of carbon dioxide and a higher global surface temperature,
might 'increase pollen quantity and induce longer pollen seasons', leading to rising levels of hay fever, eczema, and asthma.[34]
However, this possibility remains speculative; in many parts
of the world, urban expansion, the cultivation of less-prolific
pollen-producing plants, the deleterious effect of pollution
on plant life and shifting agricultural practices may well have
reduced, rather than increased, exposure to allergenic pollen.

As a result of uncertainties about the impact of outdoor pollutants and pollen, many clinicians and scientists increasingly
turned to factors in the indoor environment and Western lifestyles in order to explain global trends in asthma. Dust had been
recognized as a prominent trigger of asthma attacks by most
medical writers from the late seventeenth century. During the
Industrial Revolution, exposure to dust in factories and mines
resulted in many workers developing asthma, as well as other
forms of respiratory disease such as silicosis and asbestosis. As
occupational exposure to dangerous dusts was gradually limited by legislative measures during the nineteenth and twentieth centuries, clinical interest began to focus more closely on

house dust, which was a mixture of human and animal danders, feathers, bacteria, moulds, algae, and the remains of food, insects, and plants. Many of these substances were known to be capable of inducing allergic reactions and provoking asthma, rhinitis, and eczema.

During the 1920s, a German physician, Hermann Dekker, had speculated that the proliferation of microscopic mites in bedding might be responsible for asthma. Dekker's suspicions were eventually confirmed in the 1960s by Reindert Voorhorst and his colleagues in the Department of Allergology at Leiden. Drawing on earlier investigations by Willem Storm van Leeuwen (1882–1933), who had advocated the use of an 'allergen-proof' chamber to treat asthmatics and who had described allergic asthma in farmers exposed to mite-infested grains, Voorhorst not only demonstrated a close correlation between dust-induced allergies and specific skin reactivity to the European house dust mite *Dermatophagoides pteronyssinus*, but also established the role of temperature and humidity in determining the concentration of mites in house dust.[35] Subsequent identification of a potent allergen in mite excretion products stimulated global research into the biology and ecology of house dust mites and offered a possible explanation for modern trends in asthma.

As studies in the 1960s and 1970s suggested, fluctuations in mite populations could account for higher levels of asthma in children born during the late summer months, as mite levels were rising, and for the exacerbation of symptoms during the autumn. The regional distribution of asthma was also traced to the effect of specific climatic conditions on mites. Both the prevalence of 'climate asthma' in certain coastal regions of South Africa and the increased incidence of asthma in damp houses situated near rivers were explained in terms of the

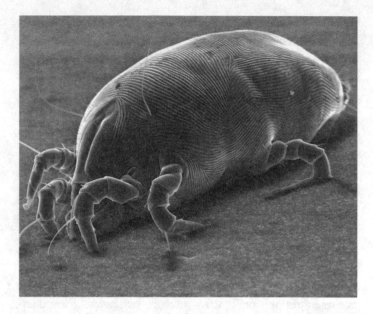

14. Scanning electron micrograph of an American house dust mite. (*Kind permission of Glen Needham, Acarology Laboratory, The Ohio State University, Columbus, Ohio*)

regional variations in humidity, which encouraged the proliferation of mites in those locations.[36] Conversely, improvements in asthmatic symptoms at high altitude were related to lower levels of house dust mites in conditions of low temperature and low humidity. In addition, while regular bed cleaning was promoted as a means of reducing mite populations, it was also recognized that bed-making constituted an occupational hazard for cleaners and housewives, thereby helping to explain the higher prevalence of mite sensitization and asthma in women.

One of the principal attractions of the house dust mite theory, however, lay in its ability to explain shifting global patterns

of asthma across time. As evidence for the role of mites in allergies deepened, clinicians began to explore the possibility that
modern domestic fashions might be driving rising trends in
asthma. During the late twentieth century, the use of fitted carpets increased dramatically, particularly in those countries that
experienced a surge in asthma morbidity and mortality, such as
New Zealand and Britain; for example, by 2000 approximately
98 per cent of British homes had fitted carpets compared with 16
per cent in France. At the same time, the composition of carpets
and other home textiles was transformed by the introduction
of artificial fibres, by the use of tufted instead of woven carpets,
and by manufacturers' attempts to design carpets in which the
dirt and dust sank to the lower layers, thereby maintaining the
floor's clean surface appearance. These developments rendered
modern carpets more resistant to vacuum cleaning, facilitated
the retention of water at the base of the pile or in the underlay,
and increased the survival and propagation of house dust mites.
By the turn of the millennium, researchers estimated that as
many as 100,000 mites might live in one square metre of carpet
and that mite allergen levels in carpets could be between six and
fourteen times higher than those on smooth floors.[37]

The proliferation of house dust mites in modern homes was
encouraged by broader political and economic factors. In the
mid-1970s, the Organization of Petroleum Exporting Countries
(OPEC) dramatically increased the price of oil in an attempt to
exert pressure on the West following the outbreak of war in
the Middle East. Faced by rising fuel costs and rampant inflation, householders in many developed, temperate countries
attempted to conserve energy and reduce heating bills by install-
ing insulation, replacing older windows with double-glazing,
and endeavouring to prevent draughts around doors. These

alterations in home design decreased ventilation, increased humidity, and provided a convenient environment for mites to thrive in carpets, bedding, and other soft furnishings, thereby promoting exposure to domestic allergens and fuelling the rise of asthma amongst modern Western populations.

Other lifestyle factors have been implicated in rising trends in asthma. In the 1980s, David Strachan, an epidemiologist at the London School of Hygiene and Tropical Medicine, proposed what later became known as the 'hygiene hypothesis' to explain the global pattern of allergic diseases. Based on an extensive study of the epidemiology of hay fever and eczema, Strachan noted that the prevalence of hay fever was indirectly related to family size: the fewer the number of siblings, the higher the prevalence of allergies.[38] Subsequent studies suggested a possible mechanism for Strachan's findings: low levels of early childhood infections, brought about by greater hygiene and fewer contacts with siblings and other children, were thought to result in imbalances in the immune system (such as the polarization of T-cell subsets towards T_H2 responses) and the production of immature immunological reactions to potential allergens, such as the house dust mite and pollen. Although not universally accepted, the hygiene hypothesis and the related concept of 'skewed antigen exposure' received speculative support from elsewhere. Studies of children in day-care nurseries and of families following anthroposophic (or more 'natural') lifestyles suggested that childhood infections and, more arguably, the avoidance of antibiotics and vaccinations might protect against the later development of asthma and other allergies.[39]

Arguments indicting Western lifestyles identified further possible causes of the increased prevalence and severity of asthma in modern populations. After the Second World War, a number of studies attempted to determine whether substantial changes in Western diets might be responsible for rising levels of allergic diseases. Research focused not only on the role of well-recognized allergens, such as eggs, milk, and wheat, but also on the introduction of a richer, more varied cuisine that exposed people to relatively new or exotic foods, such as peanuts and kiwi fruit, and on the growing popularity of pre-packed meals and 'junk food' containing high levels of salt and artificial additives. An investigation in Saudi Arabia revealed that 'asthmatic symptoms [were] 2–3 times more common in a developed urban environment than in rural villages'. According to the authors of the report, the explanation for this urban–rural gradient lay in a shift in dietary practices, away from a reliance on fresh, local produce towards the widespread consumption of 'western-type frozen and prepared foods'.[40]

Changing indoor and outdoor environments, hygiene, and diet might all have contributed to modern trends in asthma. It is also possible that alterations in working environments, and particularly contact with new chemicals, have driven rising levels of asthma. As Paul Blanc has argued, the inhalation of a number of hazardous fumes has been connected to the development of adult-onset asthma in workers. Chlorine and chloramine in swimming pools, sewage plants, and pulp paper mills, leading to the identification in 1985 of a new syndrome, reactive airway dysfunction syndrome (RADS); and cyanoacrylate instant glues, responsible for outbreaks of asthma amongst dental technicians and orthopaedic doctors and nurses exposed to methyl methacrylate in surgical cements. Recent estimates suggest that, in industrialized countries, 'one in every ten cases of asthma with onset in adulthood has a link to workplace exposures. Isocyanate-induced asthma has become the leading single cause of this occupationally related disease.'[41]

In an attempt to explain rising global trends in asthma, epidemiologists have considered other features of modern lifestyles: shifting patterns of breast-feeding, rising levels of obesity and stress, and the overuse of certain medicines have all possibly fuelled the proliferation of allergies and asthma. According to an ISAAC report published in 2008 for example, paracetamol exposure during infancy increased 'the risk of developing asthma' in childhood.[42] These putative links between lifestyle and asthma have encouraged speculations about the harmful impact of modern civilization on health. For some commentators, the explosion of asthma should serve as a warning to capitalist, consumer societies to curb the environmental destruction that accompanies unsustainable industrial and commercial expansion: like the canaries used by miners to alert them to the presence of poisonous gases, people with asthma supposedly highlight the potential hazards of irresponsible modernization.

In some ways, current concerns about the modern environmental and lifestyle determinants of asthma echo earlier twentieth-century perceptions of allergies as the exclusive preserve of the privileged and civilized elite. Historically, asthma and other allergic conditions do appear to have affected populations in the developed industrial world more frequently and more severely than those in developing countries, and to have afflicted the prosperous middle classes more often than the working classes. At the same time, images of asthma and hay fever as aristocratic diseases of civilization persisted well into the twentieth century, reinforced by occasional attempts to link asthma to social success or to intellectual and artistic creativity.

15. Asthma mortality according to social class. (*Crown copyright, reproduced from the Lung and Asthma Information Agency Factsheets 97/3 and 2001/1, http://www.sghms.ac.uk/depts/laia/laia.htm*)

However, at the dawn of the twenty-first century, the social geography of asthma has been transformed and the class gradient reversed. Although the correlation between socioeconomic status and asthma remains contested, there is some evidence to suggest that both asthmatic symptoms (particularly wheezing) and mortality from asthma have become more prominent amongst lower social classes and that the burden of asthma in the developing world is deepening. While researchers continue to focus on genetic factors, environmental pollution, indoor allergens, diet, and hygiene in an attempt to explain modern trends, the shifting social distribution of asthma reinforces the findings from episodes of asthma mortality in North America during the post-war years: like many chronic diseases, asthma now constitutes a disease of poverty, rather than one of affluence.

Asthma and industry

As mortality and morbidity rates rose after the Second World War, both the direct and indirect economic costs of asthma increased significantly. By the early 1990s, the cost of prescriptions for asthma in Britain was £347 million, a figure that constituted 11 per cent of the total National Health Service (NHS) prescription cost. At the turn of the millennium, the estimated annual cost to the NHS of treating asthma was about £850 million; by 2004, it exceeded £1 billion. However, the indirect costs of asthma from lost productivity and social security payments were thought to be even greater. In 1977, the Asthma Research Council suggested that over two million days were lost each year through asthma, 'costing more than £2 million in sickness benefits'.[43] By the 1990s, the level of certified incapacity from asthma had risen to over ten million days per year, and by 2000 the combination of lost productivity and benefits accounted for over 60 per cent of the total cost of asthma to the nation. Although comparison between countries proved difficult because of the operation of different health-care systems and different modes of calculation, similarly spiralling patterns of both direct and indirect costs were reported in North America and in many continental European countries during the last quarter of the twentieth century.

The mounting cost of asthma was attributable not only to rising levels of the disease but also to shifting approaches to management. In Britain, widespread public and professional concern about the personal and economic impact of asthma led to the establishment of dedicated asthma clinics and intensive care services and promoted the development and adoption of facilities for self-monitoring and treating asthma at home. In addition, suspicions that many asthmatics were still not receiving adequate treatment prompted the National Asthma Campaign (now Asthma UK) to devise an Asthma Charter. First published on World Asthma Day in May 2003, the Asthma Charter set out the level of care to be expected under the NHS. National guidelines for the treatment of asthma, first formulated by the British Thoracic Society in 1990, set out protocols for diagnosing and assessing children and adults with asthma, advocated a stepwise approach to treatment, established the criteria for emergency admission, and suggested standards for the organization and delivery of patient care and education. In 1991, the American National Heart, Lung, and Blood Institute published similar guidelines for the diagnosis and management of asthma as part of a National Asthma Education Program.

As asthma emerged as a global socioeconomic and public-health problem during the late twentieth century, it also paradoxically created commercial opportunities for the pharmaceutical, cleaning, food, and cosmetics industries. Pharmaceutical firms had been producing medicines to relieve asthma and other respiratory disorders from the late nineteenth century. During the middle decades of the twentieth century, both European and American companies had developed and marketed a range of anti-asthma remedies, such as the methyl xanthines, ephedrine, oral steroids, antihistamines, and non-selective bronchodilators such as isoprenaline. In the decades following the Second World War, further pharmaceutical innovations were stimulated by clearer understandings of the biological mechanisms, and particularly the inflammatory processes, involved in acute and chronic asthma: the identification of IgE in 1967 as the 'reaginic antibody' responsible for allergic reactions; growing appreciation of the cascade of intercellular mediators, such as the interleukins and leukotrienes, responsible for orchestrating immune responses and implicated in bronchial inflammation; and, more recently, an awareness that asthma is not simply an inflammatory disease but also one possibly marked by disordered repair of the bronchial wall.

During the 1960s and 1970s, a number of pivotal pharmacological developments helped to transform the lives of asthmatics. The Scottish pharmacologist Sir David Jack and his colleagues at Allen & Hanburys played a crucial role in the formulation of new treatments. Driven partly by the wave of asthma deaths putatively linked to the overuse of non-selective bronchodilators, Jack and his colleagues attempted to develop analogues of isoprenaline that would be both more selective and longer acting. The initial outcome of laboratory research was the introduction of salbutamol, the first selective β_2-adrenergic bronchodilator. Marketed in 1969 as Ventolin and distributed in what has become a distinctive blue inhaler, salbutamol became 'the most used bronchodilator in the world',[44] and rapidly enhanced Allen & Hanburys' commercial standing. According to the company's own account of its development, by 1985 annual sales of Ventolin 'had reached £171m; ten years later they exceeded £500m'.[45] Although a variety of alternative longer-acting and more selective bronchodilators have been introduced in recent years, salbutamol not only remains the most commonly prescribed inhaler for the immediate control of asthma, but is also regularly administered via a nebulizer to patients both in hospital and at home.

Following the successful identification and marketing of salbutamol, Jack's team endeavoured to develop more potent topically active anti-inflammatory steroids and to design pressurized inhalers to improve drug delivery to the lungs. Successful studies of the clinical efficacy of inhaled beclomethasone diproprionate led Allen & Hanburys to market Becotide in 1972 for the prevention of asthma. Although not universally welcomed by allergists, who continued to regard specific desensitization with preparations of house dust mite or grass pollen as the first line of treatment for asthma and other allergies, inhaled steroids revolutionized the long-term management of asthma, at the same time generating substantial profits for multinational pharmaceutical companies. The scale of the financial and political interests involved in these developments is evident in disputes about the value and safety of more recent preparations, such as Advair, which combines an inhaled steroid (fluticasone) with a long-acting bronchodilator (salmeterol) and which is administered by a revolutionary breath-activated Accuhaler. Marketed in Europe and Australia as Seretide, the annual worldwide sales of Advair totalled $4.5 billion in 2004. The following year, however, sales of the drug and the shares of GlaxoSmithKline (GSK) were damaged by warnings from the Food and Drug Administration about side effects, a decision that, according to GSK, would delay effective treatment and place many patients at greater risk.[46]

In the late 1960s, the range of drugs available to asthmatics was also boosted by the introduction of sodium cromoglycate. Synthesized from a plant that contained a naturally occurring smooth muscle relaxant, khellin, and that had been used for many centuries by doctors and their patients in Eastern Mediterranean countries to treat respiratory complaints and kidney stones, the development of cromoglycate owed much to the inspiration and persistence of Roger Altounyan (1922–87), working at Bengers Research Laboratories, part of the Fisons group. Himself an asthmatic, Altounyan opted to test the ability of a range of new compounds to improve his own symptoms. After analysing nearly 100 preparations, Altounyan identified a particular biscromone, FPL 670, which effectively relaxed bronchial muscle. Applied by a modified dry-powder inhaler or Spinhaler, disodium cromoglycate was licensed as Intal in 1968. Altounyan's work not only rapidly attracted the attention of allergists and respiratory physicians, but also had a dramatic impact on the financial fortunes of Fisons. Intal became the company's leading product, generating substantial profits and encouraging the development of analogues that would treat hay fever and food allergies.

New treatments introduced during the second half of the twentieth century undoubtedly eased the symptoms of asthma; long-term treatment with inhaled steroids combined with either regular or occasional use of selective bronchodilators effectively reduced or eliminated the wheezes, nocturnal coughs, and terrifying breathlessness that had plagued previous generations of asthmatics. However, as the examples of Allen & Hanburys and Fisons demonstrate, drug treatments for asthma also carried substantial financial benefits for the pharmaceutical industry. As patients and health services struggled to stem the rising tide of asthma, profits soared. By the 1990s, the global market for anti-asthma products was estimated to be in the region of £5.5 billion per annum. In 1995, GlaxoWellcome's sales of Ventolin, Becotide, and Serevent together amounted to £1.6 billion. More significantly, annual sales were growing: in 1994, the overall sales growth in the asthma market was approximately 14 per cent, higher than the growth rate in either the cardiovascular or gastrointestinal markets. This sales momentum has continued with the introduction of further innovative approaches to management, including the launch of the leukotriene receptor antagonist, montelukast sodium (Singulair), by Merck in 1998, and the development of monoclonal anti-IgE antibodies, first marketed by Novartis as Xolair in 2003, for adolescents and adults with severe and persistent allergic asthma.[47]

One of the most troubling features of the modern history of asthma is that improved symptomatic relief and clearer guidelines for management did not result in reduced morbidity and mortality. Indeed, at least until the mid-1990s, the prevalence and severity of asthma and a range of associated allergic diseases appeared to be rising in most countries. As a report of the Royal College of Physicians pointed out in 1992, one outcome of this apparent paradox was that many British patients turned to alternative medicine for treatment: 'Although patients who consult practitioners of alternative allergy may do so by preference, it is often also because they are dissatisfied with the conventional approach to diagnosis and treatment.'[48]

During the closing decades of the twentieth century, a variety of complementary or alternative treatments were promoted for asthma. In many Eastern countries, traditional indigenous healing methods had persisted into the twentieth century in spite of the gradual encroachment of Western biomedicine: practitioners of traditional Chinese medicine continued to use acupuncture, moxibustion, and herbs to remove phlegm and relieve coughs and wheezes; in India, commercial forms of āyurvedic medicines, such as Agastya Haritakyavaleha, Swas Chintamani Ras Gold, and Vasavaleha marketed by Dabur, were regularly employed alongside modern Western remedies in the management of asthma and other respiratory conditions; and in Japan, asthmatic patients attending private kanpō clinics were prescribed herbal remedies and moxibustion.

As dissatisfaction with Western approaches to asthma spread, Eastern remedies became increasingly popular in Europe and North America, providing alternatives to the standard pharmacological methods developed by multinational pharmaceutical companies and endorsed by Western health care systems. As Tim Brookes has demonstrated in his personal exploration of asthma and its treatment, the range of unorthodox remedies available to Western consumers in the closing decades of the twentieth century was extensive and included not only traditional Chinese and Indian approaches, but also homoeopathy, reflexology, balneotherapy, yoga, hypnotism, chiropracty, naturopathy, and the adoption of additive-free diets. In addition, in a manner reminiscent of nineteenth-century formulations of climate therapy, some asthmatics, particularly those demonstrating multiple allergic sensitivities, retreated to 'safe' environments in the desert or the mountains.[49] Alternative remedies clearly had their advocates. A survey conducted by the National Asthma Campaign in the late 1990s indicated that '60% of those with moderate asthma, and 70% with severe asthma, have used complementary therapies to treat their condition'.[50]

Although fashionable, the efficacy of many complementary remedies remains unclear. Some studies have tentatively concluded that acupuncture, relaxation, breathing techniques, and yoga might be beneficial. However, according to many orthodox practitioners, further clinical trials are required in order to establish both the advantages and the risks associated with alternative therapies. The political and economic interests inherent in disputes about the relative merits of conventional Western and alternative approaches are particularly evident in discussions of a controversial treatment for asthma developed by a Russian physician, Konstantin Pavlovich Buteyko (1923–2003). During the 1950s, Buteyko proposed a new theory of asthma, according to which asthmatic symptoms were regarded primarily as the product of overbreathing; hyperventilation and the associated reduction in carbon dioxide concentrations in the blood triggered constriction of the airways, mucosal swelling, and production of mucus. The simple remedy proposed by Buteyko involved patients learning to recognize and correct their own breathing patterns.

Scientific trials and patient testimonials have occasionally suggested that asthmatic patients can benefit from the Buteyko method, allowing them to reduce their consumption of bron-chodilators and steroids. In some cases, the results appear to have been dramatic: in 2003, Kate Jude, who suffered from chronic asthma, testified to the manner in which the 'Buteyko Technique' had substantially altered her life, allowing her to resume many daily activities that had previously been impos-sible.[51] The precise interpretation of patient testimony, however, remains disputed. In spite of positive personal accounts, many orthodox respiratory physicians have remained unconvinced by reports of the technique's efficacy. By contrast, Buteyko prac-titioners themselves have argued that enduring doubts about the method have been related not to its clinical merits but to competing professional and political interests: 'Another major reason why the Buteyko method is not proclaimed as a success by the asthma experts is that it is a drug-free treatment, and as such it poses a serious threat to the profits of drug companies and pharmacists around the world, as well as to the reputations of doctors, hospitals and academics everywhere.'[52]

Large-scale pharmaceutical companies and alternative prac-titioners were not the only professional and industrial groups embroiled in debates about rising trends in asthma. During the late twentieth century, the detergent, food, and cosmetics industries faced growing public concerns that certain products were triggering asthma attacks in susceptible patients and pos-sibly fuelling global patterns of morbidity. Industrial and state responses to these fears certainly eased the lives of people suffer-ing from asthma and other allergies: evidence that occupational asthma and eczema were linked to long-term exposure to proteolytic enzymes in the detergent industry encouraged the development of non-biological washing powders and, in Britain, led to the introduction of regulations aimed at compensating affected workers. However, in some cases, shrewd reactions to public anxieties generated further opportunities for profit. By labelling foods more clearly and offering allergen-free products, food manufacturers and retailers exploited an expanding global market for anti-allergy and organic foods. Similarly, in response to concerns about the potential for perfumes and shampoos to provoke life-threatening allergic reactions including asthma, the cosmetics industry attempted to protect and advance its financial interests by advertising products as 'hypoallergenic' or 'dermatologically tested'.

Evidence linking asthma to house dust mites also created commercial opportunities for cleaning companies. In the 1870s, Anna and Melville Bissell had developed a carpet sweeper to remove sawdust from their crockery shop in Michigan, and in the early twentieth century Hoover's production of the first electric vacuum cleaner had initially been driven by James Murray Spangler's efforts to find a solution to his dust-induced occupational asthma. Later in the century, as the role of dust mites in asthma became clearer following the work of Voorhorst and others in the 1960s, a number of European and North American cleaning companies began to develop and market a variety of products designed to eliminate or reduce the presence of ubiquitous mites: vacuum cleaners with high-efficiency particulate air filters; dehumidifiers; portable air cleaners; mite-proof covers for mattresses, pillows and duvets; and sprays used directly to kill the mites.

Approaches to asthma control that relied on removing dust mites were approved in some European countries, where barrier covers for furniture were made available through health care providers, but their legitimacy as medical products was challenged in Britain. In spite of reservations about their efficacy, however, consumers continued to purchase expensive vacuum cleaners and other cleaning commodities privately, thereby sustaining a profitable market in anti-asthma devices. The popularity of technological solutions of this nature was satirized in modern fiction. The subplot of Mark Wallington's *Happy Birthday Shakespeare* traces the attempts of a door-to-door salesman to convince the parents of an asthmatic child to invest in a new, state-of-the-art vacuum cleaner:

> A half-page advert for Turbo Vac vacuum cleaners caught my attention. *Three million dust mites live in the average mattress,* it warned. *You swallow three this size every day!* And there was a photograph of a family of fat tics magnified 438 times so they looked the size of Volkswagens. *Call Turbo Vac today and let its unique filtration system help you in your battle against allergens.*[53]

In addition to addressing contemporary fears about the rising prevalence of asthma, improved cleaning technologies exploited modern commitments to creating hygienic homes. Ironically, although driven by a desire to reduce allergen exposure, the pursuit of cleanliness in this way might have contributed indirectly to the explosion of asthma and other allergies in the decades following the Second World War: according to the hygiene hypothesis, it is likely that the trend towards smaller families living increasingly sedentary lifestyles in germ-free sanitized homes has served to prevent the spread of early childhood infections that encourage immunological maturity and protect against biological aberrations such as allergies and autoimmunity. Although the validity of this particular hypothesis remains contested, it highlights the contradictions and complexities, as well as the financial incentives, involved in trying to unravel and reverse modern patterns of asthma morbidity and mortality.

As we have seen, modern scientific narratives of asthma constituted a stark contrast to earlier medical accounts. Following a trend set by Joan Baptista van Helmont and John Floyer in the seventeenth century, most early modern medical writers on asthma revealed their own experiences of the condition in order faithfully to convey the symptoms, periodicity, prognosis, and treatment of the disease. In medical texts, such intimate confessions of respiratory infirmity provided readers with critical evidence of clinical expertise. As the anonymous author of *Instant Relief to the Asthmatic* put it in 1774:

> To understand well and to study any one disease, its progression, its operations, its different stages, and the action of various remedies on it, is the most certain means of discovering the cause and the cure: And who can have so *practical* an opportunity of doing this as the afflicted party himself?...I say, such a person, with a common share of understanding, has a *real*, others only a *general, hypothetical* knowledge of the disorder;—and this is the author's case.[54]

Personal knowledge and understanding of disease continued to shape clinical initiatives and medical writing on asthma through the nineteenth and early twentieth centuries. In the 1860s, Henry Hyde Salter based his account of asthma on his own experiences as well as on those of his patients. Similarly, in an article on asthma published in the *Lancet* in 1921, Arthur Hurst self-consciously echoed Floyer's much earlier references to the benefits generated by a physician's private knowledge of illness: 'Like Sir John Floyer...I myself suffer from asthma, so I have the advantage, which few writers on the subject possess, of 27 years of observation on my own corpus vile.'[55]

From the late nineteenth century, however, both personal narratives of disease and the sense of identity and meaning often previously shared by doctor and patient were increasingly marginalized. At one level, the rise of medical statistics, epidemiology and the randomized controlled trial promoted quantitative accounts of disease that charted levels of morbidity and mortality in whole populations: the modern significance of asthma was thus increasingly measured, by the medical profession at least, by its national or global prevalence and fatality rate rather than by its existential impact on individual patients and their families. At another level, the emergence of novel biomedical sciences, such as bacteriology, immunology, and genetics, focused medical eyes more closely on the inter- and intra-cellular pathways that were thought to initiate and moderate the pathology of asthma: individual experiences of the breathlessness and despair induced by an asthma attack were submerged under a figurative deluge of universal immunological aggressors, such as antibodies, mast cells, and inflammatory mediators.

Modern, essentially depersonalized, medical narratives of asthma were not without their successes. Careful measurement and analysis of the wave of asthma deaths amongst young people in the early 1960s in Britain not only generated a clearer understanding and awareness of the potential severity of asthma but also initiated novel public health measures that improved patient access to emergency services. Equally, greater knowledge of the molecular processes involved in allergic reactions led directly to the development of new therapies that substantially reduced the symptomatic discomfort of asthmatic patients. Recent figures suggest that those developments eventually began to reverse the rising trends in asthma experienced through the late twentieth century; from the mid-1990s, both the frequency of acute asthma episodes and mortality rates from asthma fell in many countries that had previously experienced dramatically rising trends in asthma.[56]

There were downsides to the dominance of biomedical and statistical approaches to asthma. As Tim Brookes has claimed, scientific accounts of asthma not only failed to resolve critical uncertainties about the condition but also arguably served to distance doctors from the personal experiences of patients with chronic disease.[57] In controversial cases, such as asthma associated with total allergy syndrome or multiple chemical sensitivity, traditional Western medicine was unable to explain or treat the symptoms effectively. Yet, as the language and concepts of biomedicine retreated from closer engagement with the lives of patients, the intimate biography of asthma surfaced in alternative, sometimes subversive, cultural forms at the turn of the millennium. In 1981, the English punk rock band The Toy Dolls released 'I've got asthma', during performances of which the lead singer would collapse in a fit of coughing before gasping out the final refrain. The lyrics captured the suffocating pressure of an asthma attack: 'I've got asthma and I can not breathe | can't breathe at all! | I've got an inhaler with me | I am choking and my face is blue | blue and it's getting worse!'[58] In 1995, the experimental electronic music of Aphex Twin memorialized the sound of inhalers in a track without words entitled 'Ventolin'.

Without quite matching Marcel Proust's finely nuanced literary treatment of asthma and other ailments in À la recherche du temps perdu, a number of modern novelists have nevertheless attempted to convey the manner in which asthma continues to impact on personal lives and to shape identities in the modern world. In 1991, Ferdinand Mount drew on his own experiences of asthma in childhood to provide the context for his novel *Of Love and Asthma*, in which asthma not only serves to set the narrator, Gus Cotton, apart from most of those around him but also functions as a barometer of individual and social susceptibility. In a short story entitled 'Chest', in which the world is enveloped by an impenetrable fog that threatens to suffocate both humans and animals, Will Self parodied, but perhaps reinforced, persistent popular beliefs in the emotional and neurotic roots of asthma: 'I fear my husband was asthmatic even before the fog, and he will let his emotions run away with him. Like all artists he is so terribly sensitive. When he gets upset...'[59]

The manner in which asthma operates as an indicator of personal, familial, and social distress, and in the process isolates sufferers, is equally evident in Sandra Scofield's *Walking Dunes* and Leif Enger's *Peace Like a River*, in which the fluctuating patterns of asthma experienced by the principal characters reflect and heighten narrative tensions. In Debbie Spring's *Breathing Soccer*, written to educate children about the condition, or in Robert Rigby's novelization of the film *Goal!*, asthma similarly signifies anxiety and social exclusion, particularly amongst young people.[60] In spite of remarkable developments in treatment and management, the modern asthmatic, like Proust a century earlier, constitutes a lonely figure.

Broader cultural and media portrayals of the personal consequences of asthma were echoed in the more sombre reflections of asthmatics in response to surveys conducted during the first decade of the twenty-first century. Launched on World Asthma Day in 2004, Asthma UK's report *Living on a Knife Edge* juxtaposed national statistics with a series of personal statements in order to highlight the debilitating and marginalizing effects of asthma. In 2008, a similar publication exposed the troubled lives of fifteen asthmatics in Scotland. Motivated by awareness of the suffering and needs of people with asthma, such reports were intended to provide a 'wake-up call to healthcare providers and government about the reality of living with severe symptoms of asthma', and to encourage greater state and charitable intervention.[61] Combined with parallel sociological and anthropological studies that have attempted to recapture lay understandings and experiences of asthma and other chronic allergies,[62] documents such as *Living on a Knife Edge* will perhaps help to re-establish closer clinical empathy with individuals, families, and communities affected by asthma. For whether its history is told in terms of numbers or in terms of individual stories of courage and resistance, modern asthma constitutes a reincarnation of the ancient Homeric struggle to breathe in the face of personal, social, and environmental turmoil.

EPILOGUE

Je suis asthme

I t was on 31 December 2005 that Conall suffered probably his worst attack of asthma. Siobhán and I had travelled with our three children, Ciara, Riordan, and Conall, from Devon to South Wales to celebrate the dawning of a new year with Siobhan's sister and her family. Within an hour or two of arriving in Porthcawl, and perhaps triggered by contact with his cousins' cats or by the excitement of the occasion, Conall was struggling to breathe. Flushed and distressed, he lay in Siobhán's arms, gasping, coughing, and wheezing. Like Seneca, Floyer, Proust, and many other asthmatics before him, Conall was temporarily consumed by asthma. As a French vernacular expression for breathlessness implies, when every respiratory

effort is focused solely on survival, illness and identity merge:
'Je suis asthme.'[1]

Relief was dispensed expertly and relatively swiftly by the
doctors and nurses in the Accident and Emergency Department
at the Princess of Wales Hospital in Bridgend. The immediate
administration of nebulized salbutamol and oral prednisolone
effectively reversed the bronchial constriction and began to
subdue the inflammatory reaction understood to be responsible for Conall's acute respiratory distress. Over the next two
hours, as the medication washed through his body, the wheezes
and coughs subsided and his energy and natural exuberance
were restored. Breathing more easily, we returned expectantly
to the family's New Year's Eve festivities.

In *Weaver's Daughter*, published in 2000, the American novelist Kimberly Brubaker Bradley explored a young girl's experiences of asthma as she grew up in the Southwest Territory,
later known as Tennessee, in the late eighteenth century. In
the author's note, Bradley claimed that, although she carefully
researched contemporary American life in order to describe the
social context accurately, she 'did not need to research the details
of Lizzy's illness. Like Lizzy, I have asthma, and I gave her my
own medical history.'[2] The implication of Bradley's approach—
namely, that the cardinal features of asthma have remained constant across time and space—is provocative. As we have seen,
at one level there is clearly some evidence to support Bradley's
position. The symptomatic expression and personal experience
of asthma appear relatively unchanged: modern asthma, like its
ancient, medieval, and early modern ancestors, is marked by a
wheeze, cough, and respiratory distress, which can be triggered
by a range of material and psychological factors. It is therefore likely that Marcel Proust and his parents, Seneca and his

correspondents, and Floyer and his patients would all immediately recognize the symptoms experienced by Conall and
understand their effect on our family.

At another level, Bradley's assertion that the defining features
of asthma can be readily transplanted from one era to another,
or from one person to another, is problematic. First, it is clear
that medical theories of asthma have changed substantially
since the term was first introduced by Homer nearly three thousand years ago. While ancient and medieval writers focused on
phlegm, early modern physicians tended increasingly to prioritize the role of nervous bronchospasm, a notion that was itself
partially displaced by preoccupations with inflammation and
allergy during the late nineteenth and early twentieth centuries.
In the decades following the Second World War, asthma came
to be understood in terms of a more complex cascade of pathological and psychological processes. Secondly, it is evident, as
John Gabbay has argued, that the social geography of asthma
has shifted across time: asthma was thought primarily to afflict
the overindulgent, sedentary, and intemperate upper classes in
the seventeenth and eighteenth centuries, the nervous Western
intellectual elite in the nineteenth century, the isolated and
allergic only child in the early twentieth century, and manual
workers and ethnic minorities living in conditions of urban
deprivation in both the developed and developing worlds in the
closing decades of the twentieth century.[3]

Bradley's transhistorical approach raises other challenges.
From a clinical perspective, it is apparent not only that asthma
presents in different ways in different patients at different
moments in time, but also that asthma attacks can be triggered
by different environmental factors in different people and that
the causes of rising trends in asthma morbidity and mortality

may vary both geographically and temporally. As a result of the heterogeneity of clinical appearances, some modern clinicians have suggested that 'asthma is unlikely to be a single disease entity', and that 'asthma as a symptom is really only the clinical manifestation of several distinct diseases'. From this perspective, according to an editorial in the *Lancet* published in 2006, the term itself is perhaps obsolete: 'Rather than confusing scientists, doctors, and patients even further, is it not time to step out of the straightjacket of a seemingly unifying name that has outlived its usefulness? The conclusion should surely be that it is best to abolish the term asthma altogether.'[4]

Although the logic of this argument is relatively compelling and although asthma remains an open category, the case for linguistic murder is overstated. The term 'asthma' continues to carry significant medical, social, and cultural meaning. In the first instance, asthma conveys the signs and symptoms of periodic respiratory distress with a convincingly sibilant onomatopoeic precision. Secondly, the term serves to connect multiple shared, if not entirely identical, experiences: patients and doctors from ancient to modern times, and from West to East, have understood, within limits, the existential significance and clinical implications of asthma, even though its definition and treatment have been in dispute. Finally, asthma has operated effectively to unite national and global organizations in their struggle to reduce the burden of ill health. Whether regarded merely as a descriptive term or conversely as a distinct disease, asthma is simply too deeply embedded in our collective historical and political consciousness to be discarded.

Although the clinical boundaries and scientific definition of asthma arguably remain as indistinct as they were in earlier times, the personal impact and socioeconomic importance of asthma in the modern world are both clear. According to the World Health Organization, there were approximately 150 million people in the world with asthma in 2004, a figure that had risen to an estimated 300 million by 2006. In addition, asthma is responsible for approximately 200,000 deaths worldwide each year. Conall was fortunate: like his siblings, he was born with mild asthma at a time and place when effective symptomatic treatments were readily available. For other asthmatics, both in the past and the present, the condition has been more disabling, less manageable, and too often fatal. If modern lifestyles continue to encourage asthma to 'keep its appointment', as Marcel Proust eloquently put it in a letter to his mother in 1902,[5] then asthma will remain a persistent global threat to the health and happiness of future populations deep into the new millennium.

GLOSSARY

AETIOLOGY the designated cause of a disease

ALLERGY a term introduced by Clemens von Pirquet in 1906 to denote any form of altered biological reactivity; the most common manifestations of allergic reactions include asthma, hay fever, eczema, and food allergies

ANAPHYLAXIS introduced by Charles Richet and Paul Portier in 1902 and meaning literally the 'absence of protection', the term 'anaphylaxis' is used most commonly to describe immediate, and sometimes fatal, allergic reactions, such as 'anaphlyactic shock'

ASTHMA a moderate to severe form of respiratory disorder characterized by wheezing, breathlessness, and a cough; referred to as *xiao chuan* in Chinese medicine, *zensoku* in Japan, and as *tamaka swasa* in Indian āyurvedic medicine

BRONCHOCONSTRICTION the contraction of airways in the lungs, which, in conjunction with inflammatory changes, produces the breathlessness and wheeze of asthma

BRONCHODILATOR a type of medication, such as salbutamol or Ventolin, which relaxes bronchial smooth muscle and facilitates breathing

CORTICOSTEROIDS a group of medicines, related to naturally occurring steroids, which possess anti-inflammatory properties; including drugs such as beclamethasone or

Becotide, corticosteroids can be administered systemically or directly to the lungs by inhaler

DYSPNOEA a broad term for all forms of breathing difficulty

EPIDEMIOLOGY the study of diseases in groups of people, or the pattern of diseases in populations

HISTAMINE an inflammatory mediator, which is stored in mast cells and is partially responsible for the clinical manifestations of asthma and other allergic reactions

HUMORAL THEORY a theory of disease, prominent in ancient and medieval times, according to which health and disease are the product of imbalances in the four humours—namely blood, phlegm, yellow bile, and black bile; in humoral terms, asthma is caused by the accumulation of excess phlegm in the lungs

ORTHOPNOEA a form of respiratory distress characterized by the need to sit or stand upright in order to breathe

PARENTECTOMY meaning literally 'cutting out the parent', parentectomy refers to the practice of removing asthmatic children from their homes in order to relieve their asthma and became popular in some countries in the decades following the Second World War

PREVALENCE the frequency of a disease, or the proportion of a population affected by a disease

PSYCHOSOMATIC MEDICINE a branch of medicine that emphasizes the close relationship between mind and body

REGIMEN a prescribed mode of living or lifestyle designed to preserve or restore health; in the ancient and medieval periods, a good regimen involved paying careful attention to what were referred to as the six 'non-naturals'—food and drink, environment, sleep, exercise, evacuations, and state of mind

STATUS ASTHMATICUS a severe and prolonged attack of asthma that can be fatal

STRAMONIUM a solanaceous plant, commonly referred to as thorn apple, the roots and stems of which were often smoked during the nineteenth and early twentieth centuries in order to relieve or prevent an asthma attack

NOTES

Prologue

1. *Marcel Proust: Letters to his Mother*, ed. and trans. George D. Painter (London, 1956), 121–4.

2. For further details of Proust's family, see G. D. Painter, *Marcel Proust* (Paris, 1979); Bernard Straus, *Maladies of Marcel Proust: Doctors and Disease in his Life and Work* (New York, 1980). His father's treatise was published as A. Proust and G. Ballet, *L'Hygiène du neurasthénique* (Paris, 1897).

3. *Letters of Marcel Proust*, ed. Mina Curtiss (London, 1950), 148, 281.

4. *Letters to his Mother*, ed. Painter, 125, 129–30; É. Brissaud, *L'Hygiène des asthmatiques* (Paris, 1896).

5. *Letters to his Mother*, ed. Painter, 175.

6. Céleste Albaret, *Monsieur Proust*, ed. Georges Belmont and trans. Barbara Bray (London, 1976), 51.

7. *Letters to his Mother*, ed. Painter, 100.

8. Julien Bogousslavsky, 'Marcel Proust's lifelong tour of the Parisian neurological intelligentsia: from Brissaud and Dejerine to Sollier and Babinski', *European Neurology*, 57 (2007), 129–36.

9. Albaret, *Monsieur Proust*, 67.

10. Diana Fuss, *The Sense of an Interior: Four Writers and the Rooms that Shaped Them* (New York, 2004), 194–5.

11. Marcel Proust, *The Way by Swann's*, trans. Lydia Davis (London, 2002), 125.

12. Marcel Proust, *In the Shadow of Young Girls in Flower*, trans. James Grieve (London, 2002), 71.

13. *Marcel Proust: Correspondance*, ed. Philip Kolb, xviii (Paris, 1990), 109.

Chapter 1

1. References to asthma in Homer's *Iliad* are found in book XV, lines 10 and 241.

2. Aeschylus, *The Persians*, line 484; Aeschylus, *Eumenides*, line 651; Aeschylus, *The Seven against Thebes*, line 393; Pindar, *Nemean Odes*, book 3, line 48, and book 10, line 74; Plato, *The Republic*, book 8, 556d, 568d.

3. Hippocrates, *On the Nature of Bones*, 13.19, cited in Spyros G. Marketos and Constantine N. Ballas, 'Bronchial asthma in the medical literature of antiquity', *Journal of Asthma*, 19 (1982), 263–9. On Hippocrates, see Helen King, 'Hippocrates of Cos', in W. F. Bynum and Helen Bynum (eds.), *Dictionary of Medical Biography* (Westport, CT, 2007), iii. 646–50; Jacques Jouanna, *Hippocrates*, trans. M. B. DeBevoise (Baltimore, 2001).

4. Hippocrates, *On the Sacred Disease*, in Robert Maynard Hutchins (ed.), *Hippocratic Writings*, trans. Francis Adams (Chicago, 1952), 154–60.

5. Hippocrates, *On Airs, Waters, and Places*, in Hutchins (ed.), *Hippocratic Writings*, 9–19. For a scholarly edition of this work, see Jacques Jouanna (ed.), *Hippocrate: Airs, eaux, lieux* (Paris, 1996).

6. Hippocrates, *Aphorisms*, section III, 22, 26, 30, section VI, 46, in Hutchins (ed.), *Hippocratic Writings*, 134–5, 140–1.

7. For parallel Latin and English versions of *De medicina*, see *Celsus: De medicina*, trans. W. G. Spencer (3 vols., London, 1953–71). This quote is in i (1971), 385. For Latin references to difficulty breathing, see i. 20, 96, 102, 130, 150, 340, 408, 424; ii (1953), 60, 72; iii (1953), 304.

8. *Celsus: De medicina*, trans. Spencer, i. 385–6.

9. *The Natural History of Pliny*, trans. John Bostock and H. T. Riley, iv (London, 1856), 252–6, 474–6, 492–3; v. 344.

10. For parallel Latin and English texts, see *Seneca: 17 Letters*, trans. C. D. N. Costa (Warminster Wilts., 1988), 34–7. See also Raphael C. Panzani, 'Seneca and his asthma: the illnesses, life, and death of a Roman Stoic philosopher', *Journal of Asthma*, 25 (1988), 163–74.

11. *Seneca*, trans. Costa, 44–55.

12. Robert T. Gunther (ed.), *The Greek Herbal of Dioscorides* (Oxford, 1934), bk. 1: *Aromatics*, 18–23, 28, 42, 51, 58, 83–4, 90.

13. Aretaeus, *On the Causes and Symptoms of Chronic Disease*, chapter XI, 'On asthma'; a translation by Francis Adams is available in Ralph H. Major, *Classic Descriptions of Disease* (Springfield, IL, 1945), 576–7.

14. Aretaeus, *On the Causes and Symptoms of Chronic Disease*, 576–7

15. An English translation of chapter XII can be found in *The Extant Works of Aretaeus, the Cappadocian*, trans. Francis Adams (London, 1856). See also Julius Rocca, 'Aretaeus of Cappadocia', in Bynum and Bynum (eds.), *Dictionary of Medical Biography*, i. 120–1.

16. J.-Ph. Derenne, A. Debru, A. E. Grassino, and W. A. Whitelaw, 'History of diaphragm physiology: the achievements of Galen', *European Respiratory Journal*, 8 (1995), 154–60; David J. Furley and J. S. Wilkie (eds.), *Galen on Respiration and the Arteries* (Princeton, 1984).

17. Armelle Debru, *Le Corps respirant: La Pensée physiologique chez Galien* (Leiden, 1996), 217–20. Galen's tripartite treatise *De difficultate respirationis*, in which he explores the features of asthma, orthopnoea, and dyspnoea, is available only in parallel Greek and Latin texts: Carolus Gottlob Kühn (ed.), *Medicorum Graecorum Opera*, vii (Lipsiae, 1824), 753–960.

18. *Galen: On the Affected Parts*, trans. Rudolph E. Siegel (Basle, 1976), 130–5.

19. Manuela Tecusan, 'Oribasius of Pergamum', in Bynum and Bynum (eds.), *Dictionary of Medical Biography*, iv. 944–5; Fielding H. Garrison, *An Introduction to the History of Medicine* (Philadelphia, 1929), 122–3.

20. *Stephanus of Athens: Commentary on Hippocrates' Aphorisms Sections III–IV*, trans. Leendert G. Westerink (Berlin, 1992), 151.

21. *Stephanus of Athens: Commentary*, trans. Westerink, 175.

22. *Stephanus of Athens: Commentary*, trans. Westerink, 193–5.

23. Max Meyerhof, 'Thirty-three clinical observations by Rhazes (circa 900 AD)', *Isis*, 23 (1935), 321–72.

24. Gholam Ali Bungay, Jabbar Mossawi, Seyed Ali Nojoumi, and Jonathan Brostoff, 'Razi's report about seasonal allergic rhinitis (hay fever) from the 10th century AD', *International Archives of Allergy and Immunology*, 110 (1996), 219–24.

25. For Maimonides's references to al-Rāzī, see Gerrit Bos (ed.), *Maimonides: On Asthma* (Provo, UT, 2002), 67, 84, 87, 109.

26. For an English version of Ibn Sarabyoun's work, see Luke Demaitre, 'Straws in the wind: Latin writings on asthma between Galen and Cardano', *Allergy and Asthma Proceedings*, 23 (2002), 59–93.

27. For a translation of Ibn Sīnā's writings on asthma, see Demaitre, 'Straws in the wind'. See also Nikolaj Serikoff, 'Ibn Sina', in Bynum and Bynum (eds.), *Dictionary of Medical Biography*, v. 1156–9.

28. Bos (ed.), *Maimonides: On Asthma*, 2.

29. Bos (ed.), *Maimonides: On Asthma*, 5.

30. Bos (ed.), *Maimonides: On Asthma*, 9.

31. Bos (ed.), *Maimonides: On Asthma*, 8–36 *passim*.

32. Bos (ed.), *Maimonides: On Asthma*, 37–9.

33. Bos (ed.), *Maimonides: On Asthma*, 40–58.

34. Bos (ed.), *Maimonides: On Asthma*, 44, 49.

35. Bos (ed.), *Maimonides: On Asthma*, 63.

36. Bos (ed.), *Maimonides: On Asthma*, 69, 73.

37. Demaitre, 'Straws in the wind'.

38. *The Papyrus Ebers: The Greatest Egyptian Medical Document*, trans. B. Ebbell (Copenhagen, 1937), 67. For an alternative reading, see *The Papyrus Ebers: Translated from the German Version*, trans. Cyril P. Bryan (London, 1930).

39. *The Papyrus Ebers*, trans. Ebbell, 64; Meyerhof, 'Thirty-three clinical observations', 345–6.

40. Sheldon G. Cohen and Max Samter (eds.), *Excerpts from Classics in Allergy* (Carlsbad, 1992), 2–3.

41. F. Estelle R. Simons (ed.), *Ancestors of Allergy* (New York, 1994), 34–7; National Library of Medicine, *Breath of Life* (Washington, 1998), 5–7; K. K. Chen and Carl F. Schmidt, 'The action of ephedrine, the active principle of the Chinese drug, Ma Huang', *Journal of Pharmacology and Experimental Therapeutics*, 24 (1924), 339–57.

42. *The Yellow Emperor's Classic of Internal Medicine*, trans. Ilza Veith (Berkeley and Los Angeles, 2002), 252.

43. Giovanni Maciocia, *The Practice of Chinese Medicine* (Edinburgh, 1994), 67–91, 92–104, 105–41.

44. W. Wayne Farris, 'Diseases of the premodern period in Japan', in Kenneth F. Kiple (ed.), *The Cambridge World History of Human Disease* (Cambridge, 1993), 376–84; Margaret M. Lock, *East Asian Medicine in Urban Japan: Varieties of Medical Experience* (Berkeley and Los Angeles, 1980).

45. Lois N. Magner, 'Diseases of the premodern period in Korea', in Kiple (ed.), *The Cambridge World History of Human Disease*, 392–400.

46. Dominik Wujastyk, 'Indian medicine', in W. F. Bynum and Roy Porter (eds.), *Companion Encyclopedia of the History of Medicine*, i (London, 1993), 755–78.

47. R. Viswanathan, 'The problem of asthma', *Indian Journal of Chest Diseases*, 14 (1972), 277–89; Wujastyk, 'Indian medicine'.

48. A. L. Basham, 'The practice of medicine in ancient and medieval India', in Charles Leslie (ed.), *Asian Medical Systems: A Comparative Study* (Berkeley and Los Angeles, 1976), 18–43; Gananath Obeyesekere, 'The impact of āyurvedic ideas on the culture and the individual in Sri Lanka', in Leslie (ed.), *Asian Medical Systems*, 201–26; R. A. L. Brewis (ed.), *Classic Papers in Asthma*, ii (London, 1991), introduction.

49. Gopalakrishnan Netuveli, Brian Hurwitz, and Aziz Sheikh, 'Lineages of language and the diagnosis of asthma', *Journal of the Royal Society of Medicine*, 100 (2007), 19–24.

Chapter 2

1. Alan Wykes, *Doctor Cardano: Physician Extraordinary* (London, 1969); Charles L. Dana, 'The story of a great consultation: Jerome Cardan goes to Edinburgh', *Annals of Medical History*, 13 (1921), 122–35.

2. See, e.g., Philip Barrough, *The Method of Phisicke* (London, 1583), 64–5; Nicholas Culpeper, *Culpeper's Directory for Midwives* (London, 1662), 250–1; John Pechey, *A General Treatise of the Diseases of Infants and Children* (London, 1697), 93–8. See also Luke Demaitre, 'Straws in the wind: Latin writings on asthma between Galen and Cardano', *Allergy and Asthma Proceedings*, 23 (2002), 59–93.

3. John Dallas, 'The most famous case of asthma in Scottish history', *Journal of the Royal College of Physicians of Edinburgh*, 37 (2007), 121.

4. John Baptista van Helmont, *Oriatrike or, Physick Refined* (London, 1662), 356–7. This work was previously published in 1648 as *Ortus Medicinae*; Lawrence M. Principe, 'Joan Baptista van Helmont', in W. F. Bynum and Helen Bynum (eds.), *Dictionary of Medical Biography* (Westport, CT, 2007), iii. 626–8. For Culpeper's coltsfoot preparation, see Nicolas Culpeper, *The English Physician* (London, 1652), 63–4.

5. Van Helmont, *Oriatrike*, 357.

6. Van Helmont, *Oriatrike*, 359–68 *passim*.

7. Van Helmont, *Oriatrike*, 362.

8. Thomas Willis, *Pharmaceutice rationalis: or, the Operations of Medicines in Human Bodies*, pt. II (London, 1679), 5; Mike Hawkins, 'Thomas Willis', in Bynum and Bynum (eds.), *Dictionary of Medical Biography*, v. 1309–11.

9. Willis, *Pharmaceutice rationalis*, 82.

10. Willis, *Pharmaceutice rationalis*, 82–4.

11. Willis, *Pharmaceutice rationalis*, 85–6.

12. Willis, *Pharmaceutice rationalis*, 88.

13. John Floyer, *A Treatise of the Asthma* (London, 1698), 'The Dedication'. For further discussion of Floyer's work, see John Gabbay, 'Asthma attacked? Tactics for the reconstruction of a disease concept', in Peter Wright and Andrew Treacher (eds.), *The Problem of Medical Knowledge: Examining the Social Construction of Medicine* (Edinburgh, 1982), 23–48.

14. Floyer, *A Treatise of the Asthma*, 'To the Reader'.

15. Floyer, *A Treatise of the Asthma*, 'To the Reader'.

16. Floyer, *A Treatise of the Asthma*, 6–9.

17. Floyer, *A Treatise of the Asthma*, 12–16.

18. Floyer, *A Treatise of the Asthma*, 17–22.

19. Floyer, *A Treatise of the Asthma*, 15.

20. Floyer, *A Treatise of the Asthma*, 61–2.

21. Floyer, *A Treatise of the Asthma*, 37.

22. For Floyer's discussion of causes, see *A Treatise of the Asthma*, 63–141.

23. For Floyer's lengthy discussion of treatments, see *A Treatise of the Asthma*, 142–240.

24. For an extensive discussion of Marais's music, see Clyde Henderson Thompson, 'Marin Marais, 1656–1728' (Ph.D. thesis, University of Michigan, 1957).

25. Bernardini Ramazzini, *Diseases of Workers*, trans. W. C. Wright (New York, [1713] 1940), 227, 243.

26. Thomas Maxfield, *A Short Account of God's Dealings with Mrs Elizabeth Maxfield* (London, 1778), 23–4, 28–9.

27. Tobias Smollett, *Travels through France and Italy* (Oxford, [1766] 1907), 301, 307–8.

28. Guenter B. Risse, 'Medicine in the age of Enlightenment', in Andrew Wear (ed.), *Medicine in Society: Historical Essays* (Cambridge, 1992), 149–95.

29. Anon., *An Enquiry into the Causes of the Present Epidemical Diseases* (London, 1729), 38. On Chinese recipes for asthma, see Jean-Baptiste du Halde, *The General History of China*, iv (London, 1736), 14, 28.

30. John Hill, *The Virtues of Honey* (London, 1759), 4, 26–31.

31. William Buchan, *Domestic Medicine: or, a Treatise on the Prevention and Cure of Diseases by Regimen and Simple Medicines* (5th edn., London, 1776), introduction and pp. 441–5.

32. W. F. Bynum, 'William Cullen', *Oxford Dictionary of National Biography* (Oxford, 2004).

33. George Cheyne, *The English Malady* (London, 1733), 226–37.

34. William Cullen, *First Lines of the Practice of Physic*, iii (Edinburgh, 1784), 390.

35. Cullen, *First Lines*, 397.

36. Cullen, *First Lines*, 397–8.

37. Cullen, *First Lines*, 407–10.

38. John Millar, *Observations on the Asthma and Whooping Cough* (London, 1769).

39. Thomas Withers, *A Treatise on the Asthma* (London, 1786), pp. vii–viii.

40. Withers, *A Treatise on the Asthma*, 1–2.

41. Withers, *A Treatise on the Asthma*, 7–11.

42. Withers, *A Treatise on the Asthma*, 29.

43. Withers, *A Treatise on the Asthma*, 32–9, 42.

44. Withers, *A Treatise on the Asthma*, 58–87. On the merits of emetic tartar in asthma, see William Balfour, *Illustrations of the Power of Emetic Tartar* (Edinburgh, 1819), 192–3.

45. Withers, *A Treatise on the Asthma*, 87–124.

46. William Hey, 'Case histories in medicine and surgery in the Leeds area, 1763–1809', vol. 6 in Leeds University Library, Brotherton Special Collections, MS 628/6, pp. 2, 93–6.

47. Withers, *A Treatise on the Asthma*, 226.

48. Withers, *A Treatise on the Asthma*, 277–81.

49. Millar, *Observations*, 58–63.

50. Quoted in W. F. Bynum, *Science and the Practice of Medicine in the Nineteenth Century* (Cambridge, 1994), 30–3.

51. Robert Bree, *A Practical Inquiry into Disordered Respiration; Distinguishing, the Species of Convulsive Asthma, their Causes, and Indications of Cure* (Birmingham, 1800), pp. xiii, 3.

52. Bree, *A Practical Inquiry*, 14–30.

53. Bree, *A Practical Inquiry*, 252–2, 67–8.

54. Bree, *A Practical Inquiry*, 249–72.

55. George Lipscomb, *Observations on the History and Cause of Asthma* (Birmingham, 1800), p. iii.

56. Lipscomb, *Observations*, 23–5.

57. Lipscomb, *Observations*, 86.

58. Lipscomb, *Observations*, 99–100.

59. Rostan published an account of his studies in 1818. See Carla Keirns, 'Short of breath: a social and intellectual history of asthma in the United States' (Ph.D. thesis, University of Pennsylvania, 2004), 58.

60. R. T. H. Laennec, *A Treatise on the Diseases of the Chest and on Mediate Auscultation*, 2nd edn., trans. John Forbes (London, 1827), 408. The French first edition appeared as R. T. H. Laennec, *De l'auscultation médiate* (Paris, 1819); see ii. 75–89 for the discussion of chronic catarrh and asthma.

61. Laennec, *A Treatise*, 415.

62. Charles J. B. Williams, *Pathology and Diagnosis of Diseases of the Chest* (London, 1840); F. H. Ramadge, *Asthma, its Species and Complications, or Researches into the Pathology of Disordered Respiration* (London, 1835).

63. The letter from J. Hope, dated 4 July 1836, is in the papers of John Campbell, in the archives of the Royal College of Physicians and Surgeons of Glasgow, RCPSG 31/3.

64. *Lancet,* 31 Oct. 1840, pp. 205–7.

65. *Lancet,* 7 Nov. 1840, p. 238.

66. Henry Hyde Salter, *On Asthma: Its Pathology and Treatment* (2nd edn., London, 1868), 2.

67. Hyde Salter, 'Spasmodic asthma', *Lancet,* 1, 7 Jan. 1860, p. 12.

68. Henry Hyde Salter, *On Asthma: Its Pathology and Treatment* (London, 1860), 59–60.

69. Hyde Salter, *On Asthma,* 161–204; Hyde Salter, 'On the treatment of asthma by belladonna', *Lancet,* 1, 30 Jan. 1869, pp. 152–3.

70. *Lancet,* 1, 30 June 1860, pp. 642–3.

71. Armand Trousseau, *Lectures on Clinical Medicine,* trans. P. Victor Bazire (London, [1861] 1868).

72. Thomas Pridham, *Observations on the Results of Treatment of Nearly One Hundred Cases of Asthma* (London, 1861).

73. Paul D. Blanc, *How Everyday Products Make People Sick: Toxins at Home and in the Workplace* (Berkeley and Los Angeles, 2007), 219–21.

74. Anon., 'Communications relative to the Datura Stramonium, or Thorn-apple: as a Cure or relief of Asthma', *Edinburgh Medical and Surgical Journal,* 8 (1812), 364–7; Charles Scudamore, *Cases Illustrative of the Efficacy of Various Medicines* (London, 1830), 87.

75. The words of F. H. Ramadge in 1835, quoted in Barry E. Brenner, 'Where have we been? The history of acute asthma', in Barry E. Brenner (ed.), *Emergency Asthma* (New York, 1999), 1–31, at 7. See also Alexander Marcet, 'On the medicinal properties of stramonium', *Medico-Chirurgical Transactions,* 7 (1816), 546–75.

76. *The Times,* 29 Dec. 1841, p. 3; *The Times,* 30 Dec. 1841, p. 6; *The Times,* 31 Dec. 1841, p. 3; *The Times,* 18 Oct. 1853, p. 9; Herbert Davies, 'A course of lectures on physical diagnosis of diseases of the chest', *Lancet,* 1, 5 Jan. 1850, pp. 4–8.

Chapter 3

1. A. W. B. Simpson, 'Quackery and contract law: the case of the Carbolic Smoke Ball', *Journal of Legal Studies*, 14 (1985), 345–89; Janice Dickin McGinnis, '*Carlill* v. *Carbolic Smoke Ball Company*: influenza, quackery, and unilateral contract', *Canadian Bulletin of Medical History*, 5 (1988), 121–41. The full Court of Appeal judgment is given in *Carlill* v. *Carbolic Smoke Ball Company* (1893), 1 QB 256.

2. Anon., *Instant Relief to the Asthmatic, or Those Afflicted with Shortness of Breath* (London, 1774), 22–4, 28–9; Noel Snell, 'Inhalation devices: a brief history', *Respiratory Disease in Practice* (Summer 1975), 13–15.

3. Charles Dickens, *David Copperfield* (London, 1850), ch. 30.

4. Anon., 'Treatment of spasmodic asthma', *Lancet*, 2, 12 Sept. 1863, p. 324; for responses, see *Lancet*, 2, 26 Sept. 1863, p. 380; *Lancet*, 2, 3 Oct. 1863, p. 410; *Lancet*, 2, 10 Oct. 1863, p. 430.

5. For children admitted to Great Ormond Street with asthma and other respiratory conditions, see the searchable archival website at http://www.smallandspecial.org, accessed 17 Dec. 2007. On early twentieth-century varieties, see Barry E. Brenner, 'Where have we been? The history of acute asthma', in Barry E. Brenner (ed.), *Emergency Asthma* (New York, 1999), 1–31.

6. W. Woodward, 'Asthma and eczema', *Lancet*, 1, 14 Mar. 1868, p. 366.

7. J. B. Berkart, *On Bronchial Asthma: Its Pathology and Treatment* (3rd edn., London, 1911), 41.

8. Walter Hayle Walshe, *A Practical Treatise on the Diseases of the Lungs* (London, 1871), 549–52.

9. William Osler, *The Principles and Practice of Medicine* (4th edn., New York, 1901), 631.

10. Ian Gregg, 'Some historical aspects of asthma', *Southampton Medical Journal* (1991), 11–21.

11. Walshe, *A Practical Treatise*, 543–4.

12. J. A. Swett, *A Treatise on Disease of the Chest* (New York, 1852), 195.

13. J. B. Berkart, 'The treatment of asthma', *British Medical Journal*, 7 Aug. 1880, pp. 201–2; J. B. Berkart, 'On the nature of the so-called bronchial asthma', *British Medical Journal*, 8 Nov. 1873, pp. 537–9; Berkart, *On Bronchial Asthma*, 69–71.

14. Charles H. Blackley, *Experimental Researches on the Causes and Nature of Catarrhus Aestivus (Hay-Fever or Hay-Asthma)* (London, 1873), 182, 194.

15. Alex Sakula, 'Charcot–Leyden crystals and Curschmann spirals in asthmatic sputum', *Thorax*, 41 (1986), 503–7.

16. On Brissaud, see F. B. Michel, J. L. Pujol, J. Bousquet, and P. Godard, 'History of concepts of asthma in France', *ACI International*, 8 (1996), 67–8. Brissaud's views on asthma were published as É. Brissaud, *L'Hygiène des asthmatiques* (Paris, 1896). On Foxwell, see Tee L. Guidotti, 'Consistency of diagnostic criteria for asthma from Laënnec (1819) to the National Asthma Education Program (1991)', *Journal of Asthma*, 31 (1994), 329–38. Foxwell's views on asthma appeared in his *Essays in Heart and Lung Diseases* (London, 1895), and an obituary was published in the *British Medical Journal*, 14 Aug. 1909, pp. 425–6.

17. Osler, *The Principles and Practice of Medicine*, 628–30.

18. Sir Andrew Clark, 'Some observations on the theory of bronchial asthma', *American Journal of the Medical Sciences*, 91 (1886), 104–12; Sir Andrew Clark, 'The Cavendish Lecture on a speedy and sometimes successful method of treating hay-fever', *British Medical Journal*, 11 June 1887, pp. 1255–7; Morell Mackenzie, *Hay Fever and Paroxysmal Sneezing* (4th edn., London, 1887).

19. Mackenzie, *Hay Fever*, 10; Clark, 'The Cavendish Lecture', 1255. For Beard's American perspective, see George M. Beard, *American Nervousness: Its Causes and Consequences* (New York, 1881); Mark Jackson, *Allergy: The History of a Modern Malady* (London, 2006), 62–5, 100.

20. Clemens von Pirquet, 'Allergie', *Münchener Medizinische Wochenschrift*, 53 (1906), 1457–8; C. E. von Pirquet, *Allergy* (Chicago, 1911); Jackson, *Allergy*, 27–55.

21. S. J. Meltzer, 'Bronchial asthma as a phenomenon of anaphylaxis', *Journal of the American Medical Association*, 55 (1910), 1021–4.

22. Robert A. Cooke and Albert Vander Veer, 'Human sensitization', *Journal of Immunology*, 1 (1916), 201–305; Arthur F. Coca and Robert A. Cooke, 'On the classification of the phenomena of hypersensitiveness', *Journal of Immunology*, 8 (1923), 163–82.

23. Carl Prausnitz and Heinz Küstner, 'Studies on supersensitivity', trans. Carl Prausnitz, reproduced in P. G. H. Gell and R. R. A. Coombs, *Clinical Aspects of Immunology* (Oxford, 1963), 808–16.

24. Robert A. Cooke, 'Studies in specific hypersensitiveness: IV. New etiological factors in bronchial asthma', *Journal of Immunology*, 7 (1922), 147–78.

25. Cooke, 'Studies', 147.

26. Constantine J. Falliers, 'Arnold Schoenberg and Alban Berg: the serial music and serious asthma of two leading 20th-century composers', *Journal of Asthma*, 23 (1986), 211–17; Gregg Mitman, *Breathing Space: How Allergies Shape our Lives and Landscapes* (New Haven, 2007), 10–51.

27. Leonard Noon, 'Prophylactic inoculation against hay fever', *Lancet*, 1 (1911), 1572–3; Carla Keirns, 'Germs, vaccines and the rise of allergy', in Kenton Kroker, Jennifer Keelan, and Pauline M. H. Mazumdar (eds.), *Crafting Immunity: Working Histories of Clinical Immunology* (Aldershot, 2008), 77–103.

28. John Freeman, 'An address on toxic idiopathies', *Lancet*, 2 (1920), 229–34; John Freeman, *Hay-Fever: A Key to the Allergic Disorders* (London, 1950); Jackson, *Allergy*, 56–102.

29. 'An Asthma Research Council', *The Times*, 27 Oct. 1927, p. 9d.

30. 'Causes of asthma', *The Times*, 16 Jan. 1929, p. 9d.

31. Jackson, *Allergy*, 76–80; Sheldon G. Cohen, 'The American Academy of Allergy: an historical review', *Journal of Allergy and Clinical Immunology*, 64 (1979), 332–466.

32. Babette Smith, *Coming up for Air: A History of the Asthma Foundation of New South Wales* (Sydney, 2003).

33. M. A. Krishna Iyer, 'A note on some predisposing factors in asthma', *Indian Medical Gazette* (Jan. 1926), 18.

34. Krishna Iyer, 'A note', 18; G. Raghunatha Rao, 'Some cases of asthma', *Indian Medical Gazette* (June 1926), 287–8.

35. Hugh W. Acton and Dharmendra, 'An analysis of one hundred and fifty cases of asthma', *Indian Medical Gazette* (Apr. 1933), 185–92; Hugh W. Acton and Dharmendra, 'The Arneth count, with particular reference to its diagnostic value in asthma', *Indian Medical Gazette* (May 1933), 257–64; Hugh W. Acton and Dharmendra, 'The role of the eosinophiles in the diagnosis of spasmodic asthma', *Indian Medical Gazette* (Aug. 1933), 436–43; Hugh W. Acton and Dharmendra, 'The diagnosis of the clinical types of asthma and their causation', *Indian Medical Gazette* (Nov. 1933), 636–40.

36. Warren T. Vaughan, *Strange Malady: The Story of Allergy* (New York, 1941), 7. See also W. C. Spain and Robert A. Cooke, 'Studies in specific hypersensitiveness: XI. The familial occurrence of hay fever and bronchial asthma', *Journal of Immunology*, 9 (1924), 521–69; Warren T. Vaughan, 'Minor allergy: its distribution, clinical aspects and significance', *Journal of Allergy*, 5 (1934), 184–96; W. C. Service, 'The incidence of major allergic diseases in Colorado Springs', *Journal of the American Medical Association*, 112 (1939), 2034–7.

37. Warren T. Vaughan, *Allergy and Applied Immunology* (2nd edn., St Louis, 1934), 69.

38. John A. Murphy and E. A. Case, 'Sudden death from bronchial asthma', *Journal of Allergy*, 1 (1929), 434–63; Franciso Dias, 'A fatal case of bronchial asthma', *Indian Medical Gazette* (1935), 29; Gregg, 'Some historical aspects of asthma', 20.

39. Arthur F. Coca, Matthew Walzer, and August A. Thommen, *Asthma and Hay Fever in Theory and Practice* (Springfield, IL, 1931), 133.

40. Francis M. Rackemann, *Clinical Allergy, Particularly Asthma and Hay Fever* (New York, 1931), 342.

41. E. M. Tansey, 'Henry Dale, histamine and anaphylaxis: reflections on the role of chance in the history of allergy', *Studies in History and Philosophy of Biological and Biomedical Sciences*, 34 (2003), 455–72; M. B. Emanuel and P. H. Howarth, 'Asthma and anaphylaxis: a relevant model for chronic disease? An historical analysis of directions in asthma research', *Clinical and Experimental Allergy*, 25 (1995), 15–26; Ulrich Meyer, *Steckt eine Allergie dahinter? Die Industrialiserung von Arznneimittel-Entwicklung, -Herstellung und -Vermarktung am Beispiel der Antiallergika* (Stuttgart, 2002).

42. F. M. Rackemann, 'A clinical study of 150 cases of bronchial asthma', *Archives of Internal Medicine*, 22 (1918), 517–52; F. M. Rackemann, 'Studies in asthma: I. A clinical survey of 1074 patients with asthma followed for two years', *Journal of Laboratory and Clinical Medicine*, 12 (1927), 1185–97.

43. Rackemann, 'A clinical study of 150 cases of bronchial asthma'; Rackemann, 'Studies in asthma'; Tell Nelson, 'Constitution and allergic manifestations: I. Age–sex incidence of allergic conditions', *Journal of Allergy*, 5 (1933), 124–30.

44. H. Herxheimer, 'Atropine cigarettes in asthma and emphysema', *British Medical Journal*, 15 Aug. 1959, pp. 167–71; Alex Sakula, 'A history of asthma', *Journal of the Royal College of Physicians*, 22 (1988), 36–44; R. A. L. Brewis, *Classic Papers in Asthma*, ii (London, 1991), introduction.

45. Ferdinand Mount, *Cold Cream: My Early Life and Other Mistakes* (London, 2008), 107.

46. Tim Brookes, *Catching my Breath: An Asthmatic Explores his Illness* (New York, 1995), 36–7; K. K. Chen and Carl F. Schmidt, 'The action of ephedrine, the active principle of the Chinese drug, Ma Huang', *Journal of Pharmacology and Experimental Therapy*, 24 (1924), 339–57.

47. Jesse G. M. Bullowa and David M. Kaplan, 'On the hypodermatic use of adrenalin chloride in the treatment of asthmatic attacks', *Medical News*, 83 (1903), 787–90; S. Solis-Cohen, 'The use of adrenal substances in the treatment of asthma', *Journal of the American Association*, 34 (1900), 1164.

48. Sakula, 'A history of asthma', 42; Brewis, *Classic Papers in Asthma*, ii, introduction.

49. Brewis, *Classic Papers in Asthma*, ii, introduction; Charles May, 'History of the introduction of theophylline into the treatment of asthma', *Clinical Allergy*, 4 (1974), 211–17; George Hermann, M. B. Aynesworth, and John Martin, 'Successful treatment of persistent extreme dyspnea: "status asthmaticus"', *Journal of Laboratory and Clinical Medicine*, 23 (1937), 135–48.

50. Brewis, *Classic Papers in Asthma*, ii, introduction; E. H. Fineman, 'The use of suprarenal cortex extract in the treatment of bronchial asthma', *Journal of Allergy*, 4 (1932), 182–90; 'Controlled trial of effects of cortisone acetate in chronic asthma', *Lancet*, 2 (1956), 798–803; 'Controlled trial of effects of cortisone acetate in status asthmaticus', *Lancet*, 2 (1956), 803–6; William Brockbank, Hugh Brebner, and C. D. R. Pengelly, 'Chronic asthma treated with aerosol hydrocortisone', *Lancet*, 2 (1956), 807.

51. A. W. Frankland and R. H. Gorrill, 'Summer hay-fever and asthma treated with antihistaminic drugs', *British Medical Journal*, 4 Apr. 1953, pp. 761–4; Jackson, *Allergy*, 131–2.

52. Alexander Francis, *The Francis Treatment of Asthma* (London, 1932).

53. Asthma Research Council, *Physical Exercises for Asthma* (London, 1935); Alexander Gunn Auld, *The Nature and Treatment of Asthma, Hay Fever and Migraine* (London, 1936), 13; Dharmendra, 'Asthma', *Indian Medical Gazette* (May 1936), 279–84.

54. Harry Benjamin, *Everybody's Guide to Nature Cure* (London, 1936), 308–9.

55. Mount, *Cold Cream*, 158; Rackemann, *Clinical Allergy*, 604–7; Berkart, *On Bronchial Asthma*, 95–6.

56. Erich Wittkower, 'Studies in hay-fever patients (the allergic personality)', *Journal of Mental Science*, 84 (1938), 352–69.

57. James L. Halliday, 'Approach to asthma', *British Journal of Medical Psychology*, 17 (1937), 1–53; Arthur F. Hurst, 'An address on asthma', *Lancet*, 1 (1921), 1113–17; Sir Humphry Rolleston, *Idiosyncrasies* (London, 1927), 92–102; Horace S. Baldwin, 'Studies in the asthmatic state: I. The stimulus', *Journal of Allergy*, 1 (1929), 124–9.

58. Ethan Allan Brown and P. Lionel Goitein, 'The meaning of asthma', *Psychoanalytic Review*, 31 (1944), 299–306; Dorothy Levenson, *Mind, Body, and Medicine: A History of the American Psychosomatic Society* (American Psychosomatic Society, 1994).

59. Flanders Dunbar, *Mind and Body: Psychosomatic Medicine* (New York, 1947), 177.

60. Dunbar, *Mind and Body*, 184–90.

61. Margaret M. Lock, *East Asian Medicine in Urban Japan: Varieties of Medical Experience* (Berkeley and Los Angeles, 1980), 223.

62. Mark Jackson, '"Allergy con amore": psychosomatic medicine and the "asthmogenic home" in the mid-twentieth century', in Mark Jackson (ed.), *Health and the Modern Home* (New York, 2007), 153–74.

63. Freeman, *Hay-Fever*, 150–70.

64. Stephen Black, 'Inhibition of immediate-type hypersensitivity response by direct suggestion under hypnosis', *British Medical Journal*, 6 Apr. 1963, pp. 925–9; Stephen Black, 'Shift in dose–response curve of Prausnitz–Küstner reaction by direct suggestion under hypnosis', *British Medical Journal*, 13 Apr. 1963, pp. 990–2; Stephen Black, J. H. Humphrey, and Janet S. F. Niven, 'Inhibition of Mantoux reaction by direct suggestion under hypnosis', *British Medical Journal*, 22 June 1963, pp. 1649–52; Ethan Allan Brown, 'The treatment of bronchial asthma by means of hypnosis: as viewed by the allergist', *Journal of Asthma*, 3 (1965), 101–19.

65. M. Murray Peshkin, 'Intractable asthma of childhood: rehabilitation at the institutional level with a follow-up of 150 cases',

International Archives of Allergy, 15 (1959), 91–112; Carla Keirns, 'Short of breath: a social and intellectual history of asthma in the United States' (Ph.D. thesis, University of Pennsylvania, 2004), 182–203.

66. Brookes, *Catching my Breath*, 190.

67. Frances Wilmot and Pauline Saul, *A Breath of Fresh Air: Birmingham's Open-Air Schools 1911–1970* (Chichester, 1998), 82.

68. 'Patrick White: The Nobel Prize in Literature 1973: Autobiography', at http://nobelprize.org/nobel_prizes/literature/laureates/1973/white-autobio.html, accessed 14 July 2008.

69. 'Patrick White: The Nobel Prize in Literature 1973: Autobiography'.

70. Clarence E. De La Chapelle, 'Health in the selection of students', *American Journal of Nursing*, 41 (1941), 79–82; Cohen, 'The American Academy of Allergy', 429–31.

71. Anne Sexton, 'Man and wife', in Anne Sexton, *Live or Die* (London, 1966), 27–8. See also anon., 'Man's asthma cured by wife's death', *The Times*, 29 Mar. 1962, p. 5a; C. P. Taylor, *Allergy*, in Jim Haynes (ed.), *Traverse Plays* (London: Penguin, 1966), 104–39.

72. On Sander, see Keirns, 'Short of breath', 202–3; on health villages, see Abraham Stern, *Asthma and Emotion* (New York, 1981), 47.

Chapter 4

1. Sanjay Kumar, 'Traditional Indian remedy for asthma challenged in court', *British Medical Journal*, 328 (2004), 1457. Disputes about the fish treatment have also been covered in many Indian newspapers, including the *Deccan Chronicle*, the *Hindu*, and the *Khaleej Times*.

2. Tim Brookes, *Catching my Breath: An Asthmatic Explores his Illness* (New York, 1995), 3–4.

3. Brookes, *Catching my Breath*, 13, 283.

4. Quoted in L. A. Reynolds and E. M. Tansey (eds.), *Childhood Asthma and Beyond: Wellcome Witnesses to Twentieth Century Medicine*, xi (London, 2001), 9.

5. John Morrison Smith, 'The recent history of the treatment of asthma: a personal view', *Thorax*, 38 (1983), 244–53.

6. Ministry of Transport and Civil Aviation, *The Ship's Captain's Medical Guide* (London, 1952), 167, quoted in Reynolds and Tansey (eds.), *Childhood Asthma*, 21.

7. J. McCracken, 'A memorable patient: death in the Scottish highlands', *British Medical Journal*, 315 (1997), 408; Reynolds and Tansey (eds.), *Childhood Asthma*, 14–15.

8. John Morrison Smith, 'Death from asthma', *Lancet*, 1 (1966), 1042; F. E. Speizer, R. Doll, and P. Heaf, 'Observations on recent increase in mortality from asthma', *British Medical Journal*, 10 Feb. 1968, pp. 335–9; W. H. W. Inman and A. M. Adelstein, 'Rise and fall of asthma mortality in England and Wales in relation to use of pressurised aerosols', *Lancet*, 2 (1969), 279–85.

9. W. H. W. Inman, *Don't Tell the Patient: Behind the Drug Safety Net* (Los Angeles, 1999), 61–79. For media coverage, see 'Implications of increase in asthma deaths', *The Times*, 13 Aug. 1968, p. 7e; 'Alarm at asthma deaths', *The Times*, 28 Oct. 1968, p. 2a; 'Drug warning to asthma patients: care needed with aerosols', *The Times*, 23 June 1967, p. 3e.

10. CIBA Guest Symposium, 'Terminology, definitions, and classification of chronic pulmonary emphysema and related conditions', *Thorax*, 14 (1959), 286–99; J. G. Scadding, 'Meaning of diagnostic terms in broncho-pulmonary disease', *British Medical Journal*, 7 Dec. 1963, pp. 1425–30.

11. J. M. Perkin, 'Allergy in general practice', *Practitioner*, 208 (1972), 776–83.

12. D. J. Pereira Gray, 'Gale Memorial Lecture 1979: just a GP', *Journal of the Royal College of General Practitioners*, 30 (1980), 231–9; Roger Robinson, 'A paper that changed my practice: wheezy children', *British Medical Journal*, 302, 22 June 1991, p. 1516.

13. Speizer, Doll, and Heaf, 'Observations on recent increase', 337.

14. Speizer, Doll, and Heaf, 'Observations on recent increase', 337. See also F. E. Speizer, R. Doll, P. Heaf, and L. B. Strang, 'Investigation into use of drugs preceding death from asthma', *British Medical Journal*, 10 Feb. 1968, pp. 339–43; M. J. Greenberg, 'Isoprenaline in myocardial failure', *Lancet*, 2 (1965), 442–3; M. J. Greenberg and A. Pines, 'Pressurized aerosols in asthma', *British Medical Journal*, 4 Mar. 1967, p. 563; Bryan Gandevia, 'Pressurized aerosols in asthma', *British Medical Journal*, 13 May 1967, p. 441.

15. Neil Pearce, *Adverse Reactions: The Fenoterol Story* (Auckland, 2007); Paul Stolley, 'Why the United States was spared an epidemic of deaths due to asthma', *American Review of Respiratory Disease*, 105 (1972), 883–90; G. Keating, E. A. Mitchell, R. Jackson, R. Beaglehole, and H. Rea, 'Trends in sales of drugs for asthma in New Zealand, Australia, and the United Kingdom, 1975–81', *British Medical Journal*, 289 (1984), 348–51.

16. 'Tension blamed for Negroes' asthma', *The Times*, 26 July 1965, p. 8c; 'Five die in Cuba asthma wave', *The Times*, 27 Sept. 1963, p. 12c.

17. Gregg Mitman, *Breathing Space: How Allergies Shape our Lives and Landscapes* (New Haven, 2007), 130–66.

18. Ian Whitmarsh, *Biomedical Ambiguities: Race, Asthma, and the Contested Meaning of Genetic Research in the Caribbean* (Ithaca, NY, 2008).

19. Harvey W. Phelps, Gerald W. Sobel, and Neal A. Fisher, 'Air pollution asthma among military personnel in Japan', *Journal of the American Medical Association*, 175 (1961), 990–3; Harvey W. Phelps and Shigeo Koike, '"Tokyo–Yokohama asthma": the rapid development of respiratory distress presumably due to air pollution', *American Review of Respiratory Diseases*, 86 (1962), 55–63; Rodney R. Beard, Robert J. M. Horton, and Roy O. McCaldin, 'Observations on Tokyo–Yokohama asthma and air pollution in Japan', *Public Health Reports*, 79 (1964), 439–44; Rexford G. Haycraft, 'Tokyo–Yokohama asthma: a review and some current concepts', *California Medicine*, 105 (1966), 89–92.

20. Peng Guo, Kazuhito Yokoyama, Masami Suenaga, and Hirotaka Kida, 'Mortality and life expectancy of Yokkaichi asthma patients, Japan: late effects of air pollution in 1960–70s', *Environmental Health*, 7 (2008), available at http://www.ehjournal.net/content/7/1/8, accessed 21 Sept. 2008.

21. Quoted in John Gabbay, 'Asthma attacked? Tactics for the reconstruction of a disease concept', in Peter Wright and Andrew Treacher (eds.), *The Problem of Medical Knowledge: Examining the Social Construction of Medicine* (Edinburgh, 1982), 23–48.

22. A. E. Tattersfield, A. J. Knox, J. R. Britton, and I. P. Hall, 'Asthma', *Lancet*, 360 (2002), 1313–22.

23. J. K. Peat, B. G. Toelle, G. B. Marks, and C. M. Mellis, 'Continuing the debate about measuring asthma in population studies', *Thorax*, 56 (2001), 406–11.

24. Department of Health, *Asthma: An Epidemiological Overview* (London, 1995); Lung & Asthma Information Agency (LAIA), Factsheets 92/1, 92/4, 93/6, 95/1, 96/2, 97/3, 99/1, 2002/1, available at http://www.sghms.ac.uk/depts/laia/laia.htm, accessed 6 May 2008; D. M. Fleming and D. L. Crombie, 'Prevalence of asthma and hay fever in England and Wales', *British Medical Journal*, 294 (1987), 279–83; Mark N. Upton, Alex MacConnachie, Charles McSharry, Carole L. Hart, George Davey-Smith, Charles R. Gillis, and Graham C. M. Watt, 'Intergenerational 20 year trends in the prevalence of asthma and hay fever in adults: the Midspan family study surveys of parents and offspring', *British Medical Journal*, 321 (2000), 88–92.

25. Derek J. Chadwick and Gail Cardew (eds.), *The Rising Trends in Asthma* (Chichester, 1997); UCB Institute of Allergy, *European Allergy White Paper: Allergic Diseases as a Public Health Problem* (Brussels, 1997).

26. Ian Gregg, 'Epidemiological aspects', in T. J. H. Clark and S. Godfrey (eds.), *Asthma* (2nd edn., London, 1983), 242–83; Ian Gregg, 'Epidemiological research in asthma: the need for a broad perspective', *Clinical Allergy*, 16 (1986), 17–23; WHO, 'The prevention

of allergic diseases', *Clinical Allergy*, 16 (1986), supplement; Chadwick and Cardew (eds.), *Rising Trends*.

27. John David van Sickle, 'The rise of asthma and allergy in South India: how representations of illness influence medical practice and the marketing of medicine' (Ph.D. thesis, University of Arizona, 2004).

28. J. P. Sethi, D. P. Mathur, V. S. Baldwa, U. S. Mathur, and I. C. Sogani, 'Natural history of bronchial asthma in India', *Journal of Asthma Research*, 6 (1969), 187–97; R. Viswanathan, 'The problem of asthma', *Indian Journal of Chest Diseases*, 14 (1972), 277–89.

29. S. T. Holgate, 'Lessons learnt from the epidemic of asthma', *Quarterly Journal of Medicine*, 97 (2004), 247–57; William Cookson, 'The alliance of genes and environment in asthma and allergy', *Nature*, 402, supplement (1999), B5–11; William Cookson, *The Gene Hunters* (London, 1994), 123–42.

30. *Committee on Air Pollution—Report* (London, HMSO, 1954), paras. 12–18; Mark Jackson, 'Cleansing the air and promoting health: the politics of pollution in post-war Britain', in Virginia Berridge and Kelly Loughlin (eds.), *Medicine, the Market and the Mass Media: Producing Health in the Twentieth Century* (London, 2005), 19–41.

31. Mark Jackson, *Allergy: The History of a Modern Malady* (London, 2006), 154–66.

32. Erika von Mutius, Christian Fritzsch, Stephan K. Weiland, Gabriele Röll, and Helgo Magnussen, 'Prevalence of asthma and allergic disorders among children in united Germany: a descriptive comparison', *British Medical Journal*, 305 (1992), 1395–9.

33. A. Wardlaw (ed.), 'Air pollution and allergic disease: report of a working party of the British Society for Allergy and Clinical Immunology', *Clinical and Experimental Allergy*, 25, supplement 3 (1995), 10.

34. Paul John Beggs and Hilary Jane Bambrick, 'Is the global rise of asthma an early impact of anthropogenic climate change?', *Environmental Health Perspectives*, 113 (2205), 915–19.

35. R. Voorhorst, F. Th. M. Spieksma, H. Varekamp, M. J. Leupen, and A. W. Lyklema, 'The house-dust mite (Dermatophagoides pteronyssinus) and the allergen it produces: identity with the house-dust allergen', *Journal of Allergy*, 39 (1967), 325–39.

36. David Ordman, 'The evolution in South Africa of the concept of "climate asthma" and of the associated climate patterns', *South African Medical Journal*, 44 (1970), 1236–40; David Ordman, 'The incidence of "climate asthma" in South Africa: its relation to the distribution of mites', *South African Medical Journal*, 45 (1971), 739–43.

37. Jill Warner, *Allergic Diseases and the Indoor Environment* (London, 2000).

38. David P. Strachan, 'Hay fever, hygiene and household size', *British Medical Journal*, 299 (1989), 1259–60.

39. David P. Strachan, 'Family size, infection and atopy: the first decade of the "hygiene hypothesis"', *Thorax*, 55, supplement 1 (2000), S2–10; Tse Wen Chang and Ariel Y. Pan, 'Cumulative environmental changes, skewed antigen exposure, and the increase of allergy', *Advances in Immunology*, 98 (2008), 39–83; Claire Infante-Rivard, Devendra Amre, Denyse Gautrin, and Jean-Luc Malo, 'Family size, day-care attendance, and breast-feeding in relation to the incidence of childhood asthma', *American Journal of Epidemiology*, 153 (2001), 653–8.

40. Nariman Hijazi, Bahaa Abalkhail, and Anthony Seaton, 'Diet and childhood asthma in a society in transition: a study in urban and rural Saudi Arabia', *Thorax*, 55 (2000), 775–9.

41. Paul D. Blanc, *How Everyday Products Make People Sick: Toxins at Home and in the Workplace* (Berkeley and Los Angeles, 2007), 80–2.

42. Richard Beasley, Tadd Clayton, Julian Crane, Erika von Mutius, Christopher K. W. Lai, Stephen Montefort, and Alistair Stewart, 'Association between paracetamol use in infancy and childhood, and risk of asthma, rhinoconjunctivitis, and eczema in children aged 6–7 years: analysis from Phase Three of the ISAAC programme', *Lancet*, 372 (2008), 1039–48.

43. 'More asthma but progress towards control', *The Times*, 4 Apr. 1977, p. 2e.

44. Sir David Jack, 'Drug treatment of bronchial asthma 1948–1995— years of change', *International Pharmacy Journal*, 10 (1996), 50–2.

45. '30 years of Ventolin: text for island display, GWHW, Greenford', Allen & Hanburys' Heritage Archive. I am grateful to Sarah Flynn, archivist at GlaxoWellcome until 2000, for supplying a copy of this document.

46. Paul Durman and Dominic O'Connell, 'Glaxo hit by asthma drug ruling', *Sunday Times*, 20 Nov. 2005, Life & Style section.

47. For further discussion of pharmacological developments and their economic impact, see Jackson, *Allergy*.

48. A. B. Kay and M. H. Lessof, *Allergy: Conventional and Alternative Concepts* (London, 1992), 1.

49. Brookes, *Catching my Breath*, 181–208. The use of isolated retreats for 'total allergy syndrome' is explored in Todd Haynes's film *Safe* (1996), which is discussed in Matthew Gandy, 'Allergy and allegory in Todd Haynes' *Safe*', in Mark Shiel and Tony Fitzmaurice (eds.), *Screening the City* (London, 2003), 239–61.

50. Alyson L. Huntley, Adrian White, and Edzard Ernst, 'Complementary medicine for asthma', *Focus on Alternative and Complementary Therapies*, 5 (2000), 111–16; Roberta Bivins, *Alternative Medicine? A History* (Oxford, 2007).

51. Kate Jude's story was reported on the BBC's online news channel on Monday, 21 Apr. 2003, available at http://news.bbc.co.uk/1/hi/health/2805039.stm, accessed 17 Oct. 2008.

52. Alexander Stalmatski, *Freedom from Asthma: Buteyko's Revolutionary Treatment* (London, 1997), 13.

53. Mark Wallington, *Happy Birthday Shakespeare* (London, 2000), 1.

54. Anon., *Instant Relief to the Asthmatic, or Those Afflicted with Shortness of Breath* (London, 1774), 8–9.

55. Arthur Hurst, 'An address on asthma', *Lancet*, 1 (1921), 1113–17.

56. See, e.g., R. S. Sunderland and D. M. Fleming, 'Continuing decline in acute asthma episodes in the community', *Archives of Disease in Childhood*, 89 (2004), 282–5; H. Ross Anderson, 'Editorial: prevalence of asthma', *British Medical Journal*, 330 (2005), 1037–8; Martin Johnston, 'Asthma symptoms decline', *New Zealand Herald*, 17 Oct. 2008.

57. Brookes, *Catching my Breath*, 13.

58. The lyrics are available at the band's website, http://www. thetoydolls.com, accessed 8 Sept. 2008.

59. 'Chest', in Will Self, *Grey Area and Other Stories* (London, 2006), 143–88; Ferdinand Mount, *Of Love and Asthma* (London, 1991).

60. Sandra Scofield, *Walking Dunes* (New York, 1992); Leif Enger, *Peace like a River* (London, 2001); Debbie Spring, *Breathing Soccer* (Saskatoon, 2008); Robert Rigby, *Gaol!* (London, 2005).

61. Asthma UK, *Living on a Knife Edge* (London, 2004), 21; Asthma UK Scotland, *15 Years, 15 Stories: Asthma in Scotland – Seen through 15 Lives* (Edinburgh, 2008).

62. Sonja Olin Lauritzen, 'Lay voices on allergic conditions in children: parents' narratives and the negotiation of a diagnosis', *Social Science and Medicine*, 58 (2004), 1299–1308; Van Sickle, 'The rise of asthma and allergy in South India'.

Epilogue

1. F. B. Michel, J. L. Pujol, J. Bousquet, and P. Godard, 'History of concepts of asthma in France', *ACI International*, 8 (1996), 67–8.

2. Kimberly Brubaker Bradley, *Weaver's Daughter* (New York, 2000), 163.

3. John Gabbay, 'Asthma attacked? Tactics for the reconstruction of a disease concept', in Peter Wright and Andrew Treacher (eds.),

The Problem of Medical Knowledge: Examining the Social Construction of Medicine (Edinburgh, 1982), 23–48.

4. Anon., 'Editorial: a plea to abandon asthma as a disease concept', Lancet, 368 (2006), 705.

5. Marcel Proust: Letters to his Mother, ed. and trans. George D. Painter (London, 1956), 134–5.

FURTHER READING

The history of asthma has been relatively neglected compared with many other diseases. There are no previous extensive histories of the condition from ancient to modern times, only scattered references to asthma in standard histories of health and medicine, and few close studies of either prominent medical theories or patient experiences of asthma in historical context. Nevertheless, a number of texts offer useful starting points for the student of asthma in the past.

Several scholars have briefly summarized the history of asthma across the centuries, in the process providing some indication of the changing epidemiology and shifting medical theories of asthma. The most prominent author has arguably been Alex Sakula, whose articles have done much to promote historical interest in the condition amongst clinicians: Alex Sakula, 'A history of asthma', *Journal of the Royal College of Physicians*, 22 (1988), 36–44, and 'Charcot–Leyden crystals and Curschmann spirals in asthmatic sputum', *Thorax*, 41 (1986), 503–7. Similar overviews are also given by Ian Gregg, 'Some historical aspects of asthma', *Southampton Medical Journal* (1991), 11–21, Edmund Keeney, 'The history of asthma from Hippocrates to Meltzer', *Journal of Allergy*, 35 (1964), 215–26, and Leon Unger and M. Coleman Harris, 'Allergy and bronchial asthma', *Annals of Allergy*, 32 (1974), 214–30. An excellent German survey of clinical and scientific developments is available in Hans Schadewaldt, *Geschichte der Allergie*, ii (Munich and Diesenhofen, 1980), 183–354.

Perhaps the most constructive introduction to the broad history of asthma, however, is provided in a wonderful collection of seminal papers edited by R. A. L. Brewis. In the two volumes of *Classic Papers in Asthma* (London, 1991), Brewis not only brings together facsimile editions of many famous medical accounts of asthma through the ages, but also offers persuasive discussions of both the evolution of clinical understandings of asthma and changing approaches to treatment across time and space.

Although the condition was clearly of interest to ancient authors, such as Hippocrates, Aretaeus, and Galen, asthma figures only rarely in histories of ancient health and medicine, meriting only a brief reference, for example, in Mirko D. Grmek, *Diseases in the Ancient Greek World* (Baltimore, 1989). Some indication of ancient approaches is given by Spyros G. Marketos and Constantine N. Ballas, 'Bronchial asthma in the medical literature of Greek antiquity', *Journal of Asthma*, 19 (1982), 263–9, and Galen's understanding of respiration and respiratory diseases, including asthma, is neatly explored in the French work of Armelle Debru, *Le Corps respirant: La Pensée physiologique chez Galien* (Leiden, 1996). Seneca's experiences of asthma and various other illnesses are discussed in Raphael C. Panzani, 'Seneca and his asthma: the illnesses, life, and death of a Roman Stoic philosopher', *Journal of Asthma*, 25 (1988), 163–74. The most comprehensive account of subsequent approaches to asthma is given by Luke Demaitre, whose 'Straws in the wind: Latin writings on asthma between Galen and Cardano', *Allergy and Asthma Proceedings*, 23 (2002), 59–93, offers excerpts from, and a commentary on, medieval and early Renaissance accounts of the condition. The work of Maimonides in particular is explored constructively in the introduction and notes in Gerrit Bos (ed.), *Maimonides: On Asthma* (Provo, UT, 2002).

Early modern formulations of asthma have attracted even less attention from historians of medicine than ancient asthma. There is a brief discussion focusing on the works of van Helmont, Willis, and Floyer in R. Ellul-Micallef, 'Asthma: a look at the past', *British Journal of Diseases of the Chest*, 70 (1976), 112–16, and a useful account of the theories and experiences of famous eighteenth- and nineteenth-century asthmatics, including the clinicians John Millar, Robert Bree, Thomas W. King, Henry Hyde Salter, and Morrill Wyman, in Sheldon G. Cohen, 'Asthma among the famous', *Allergy and Asthma Proceedings*, 17 (1996), 161–74, and 18 (1997), 251–68. The only critical analysis of early modern asthma, however, is an excellent essay by John Gabbay, focusing on the writings of John Floyer. In 'Asthma attacked? Tactics for the reconstruction of a disease concept', in Peter Wright and Andrew Treacher (eds.), *The Problem of Medicine Knowledge: Examining the Social Construction of Medicine* (Edinburgh, 1982), 23–48, Gabbay makes a convincing argument for carefully situating historical writings on asthma, and indeed other disease categories, within particular socio-political contexts, rather than analysing and evaluating them from a modern, presentist, perspective.

Clinical understandings of asthma from the late nineteenth through the twentieth century were largely preoccupied with the role of allergy. Extensive discussions of asthma within this context are evident in several recent studies, such as the magnificent analysis of American allergies in Gregg Mitman, *Breathing Space: How Allergies Shaped our Lives and Landscapes* (New Haven, 2007), and the account of global trends in allergic diseases in Mark Jackson, *Allergy: The History of a Modern Malady* (London, 2006). More directly, Carla Keirns's doctoral dissertation 'Short of breath: a social and intellectual history of asthma in the

United States' (University of Pennsylvania, 2004) provides an original and carefully evidenced history of medical approaches and patient experiences of asthma in modern America. Keirns's work was instrumental in the genesis of an exhibition on the history of asthma at the National Library of Medicine between 1999 and 2001, which was accompanied by an educational booklet, *Breath of Life* (National Library of Medicine, 1999).

Insights into modern trends in asthma morbidity and mortality are more readily gained from epidemiological, than historical, studies. Particularly useful overviews of global trends are given in the various contributions to Derek J. Chadwick and Gail Cardew (eds.), *The Rising Trends in Asthma* (Chichester, 1997), and in Ian Gregg, 'Epidemiological aspects', in T. J. H. Clark and S. Godfrey (eds.), *Asthma* (2nd edn., London, 1983), 242–83. John David van Sickle's doctoral dissertation 'The rise of asthma and allergy in South India: how representations of illness influence medical practice and the marketing of medicine' (University of Arizona, 2004) offers an interesting alternative non-Western perspective on modern trends. Of course, accurately identifying patterns of disease across time has always been dependent on diagnostic criteria, which in relation to asthma have remained contested in the modern period. Shifting approaches to diagnosing asthma are explored in a review article by Tee L. Guidotti, 'Consistency of diagnostic criteria for asthma from Laënnec (1819) to the National Asthma Education Program (1991)', *Journal of Asthma*, 31 (1994), 329–38.

Another prominent feature of asthma during the twentieth century has been the remarkable development of novel pharmaceutical treatments. Perceptive reflections on changing treatment options are provided by a number of clinicians looking back at their own practice or reviewing the history of specific technologies, particularly: John Morrison Smith, 'The recent history of the treatment of asthma: a personal view', *Thorax*, 38 (1983), 244–53; David Jack, 'Drug treatment of bronchial asthma 1948–95—years of change', *International Pharmacy Journal*, 10 (1996), 50–2; and Jean-François Dessanges, 'A history of nebulization', *Journal of Aerosol Medicine*, 14 (2001), 65–71. More expansive reflections are provided by the contributors in L. A. Reynolds and E. M. Tansey (eds.), *Childhood Asthma and Beyond: Wellcome Witnesses to Twentieth Century Medicine* (London, 2001).

While the history of asthma can certainly be told in terms of official statistics, shifting medical knowledge and practice, and changing public representations, it can also be accessed through the experiences of asthmatics such as Marcel Proust, whose life provides the structural foundations for this book. Proust's many illnesses are explored in Bernard Straus, *Maladies of Marcel Proust: Doctors and Disease in his Life and Work* (New York, 1980), in Céleste Albaret, *Monsieur Proust*, ed. Georges Belmont and trans. Barbara Bray (London, 1976), and more briefly in Constantine J. Falliers, 'The literary genius and the many maladies of Marcel Proust', *Journal of Asthma*, 23 (1986), 157–64. However, the acute respiratory and psychological distress precipitated by asthma is particularly evident in Proust's letters to his mother and friends, available in *Letters of Marcel Proust*, ed. Mina Curtiss (London, 1950), and *Marcel Proust: Letters to his Mother*, ed. and trans. George D. Painter (London, 1956). Close study of such intimate documents of despair reveals the colossal impact of asthma on people in all places and at all times.

INDEX

Note: page numbers in *italic* refer to illustrations.